Health Care Turning Point

Health Care Turning Point

Why Single Payer Won't Work

Roger M. Battistella

The MIT Press
Cambridge, Mass.
London, England

For information about special quantity discounts, please email special_sales@mitpress .mit.edu

This book was set in Palatino by Graphic Composition, Inc. Printed and bound in the United States of America.

Library of Congress Cataloging-in-Publication Data

Battistella, Roger M.
Health care turning point : why single payer won't work / Roger M. Battistella.
    p. ; cm.
Includes bibliographical references and index.
ISBN 978-0-262-01407-6 (hardcover : alk. paper)
1. Medical policy—United States. 2. Health care reform—United States. I. Title.
[DNLM: 1. Health Care Reform—United States.   WA 540 AA1 B336h 2010]
RA395.A3B285   2010
362.1'0425—dc22
                                                        2009033439

10   9   8   7   6   5   4   3   2   1

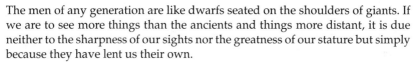

The men of any generation are like dwarfs seated on the shoulders of giants. If we are to see more things than the ancients and things more distant, it is due neither to the sharpness of our sights nor the greatness of our stature but simply because they have lent us their own.

—Bernard of Chartres

To my mother who sacrificed for a dream—
I hope I have made her proud.

Contents

Acknowledgments

Writing a book is a lonely activity in which the intellectual perseverance and discipline required misleads one into exaggerating the accomplishment of individual effort when, truth be told, the outcome represents the contributions of numerous past and present influences. I am pleased to acknowledge some of my more recent influences. First are my faculty colleagues in the Sloan Graduate Program in Health Administration and Policy program at Cornell who either provided encouragement in the conceptual and proposal stages, read and commented on early chapter drafts, or helped to track down references. They include Professors John Kuder, Will White, and Sean Nicholson.

Colleagues from other universities who provided encouragement and support during the proposal stage include Regina Herzlinger, the Nancy R. McPherson Professor of Business Administration, Harvard Business School; Jim Begun, the James A. Hamilton Professor of Health Care Management, School of Public Health, University of Minnesota; and Tom Rundall, the Henry Kaiser Professor of Organized Health Systems Research and Director, Center for Health Management Research School of Public Health, University of California, Berkeley.

My indebtedness extends to David N. Gans, PhD, Vice President, Practice Management Resources, Medical Group Management Association, for providing data on the economics and organization of physician practices; Mark Pauly, PhD, Professor of Health Care Management, The Wharton School, University of Pennsylvania, for useful suggestions on calculating changes in the size of the private-pay health care market; and Alicia H. Munnell, PhD, Director, Center for Retirement Research, Boston College, for guiding me to information on the size of state and local government unfunded retiree health obligations. Alan Stoll, Emeritus Administrator and Vice President, Fallon Clinic, Worcester, Massachusetts, and current Vice President, Pivott Health, provided helpful research leads and suggestions, as well as encouraging me to persist in completing the manuscript. My gratitude extends to Thomas P. Weil, PhD, a valued friend and collaborator since our long ago doctoral student days at the University of Michigan, School of Public Health. Tom, in the course of his pre-retirement career as an educator and health and hospital services consultant, never tired of reminding me that the true test of the value of theory is in its practical application and, based on his own experience with book publishing, provided sound advice on how to expedite the process. Sam Levey, PhD, the Gerhard Hartman Professor of Health Management and Policy, School of Public Health, University of Iowa, is another colleague and friend who helped to ease the way in my taking on this project.

Thanks further to the administrative support staff in Cornell's Department of Policy Analysis and Management who assisted me in dealing with word processing glitches and project correspondence: Lois Brown, Debbie Perlmutter, and Angelica Hammer. I am also grateful to the staff of Cornell's excellent library system. They assisted me in navigating electronic access to reference materials without having to leave my office. All of whom I dealt with were unfailingly courteous, and helpful.

Several persons rank especially high in the gratitude category. They include Jeanne Schmidlin, whom I depended on to catch and correct errors of grammar and punctuation and who astutely noted content requiring clarification and amplification, and John S. Covell, Senior Editor, Economics, Finance, and Business, MIT Press. Without his endorsement and support, this book, which struck others as uncomfortably heretical in the challenge it poses to the conventional wisdom, possibly would not have been published. And to Paul King who, in addition to tutoring me in the mysteries of the digital age and responding to urgent appeals for help in correcting word processing mishaps arising from my inexperience in anything more complicated than email, relieved me of my responsibilities in the family business, a boutique winery where I am in charge of the winemaking and vineyard management, so that I could concentrate on completing this manuscript.

Finally, there is my beautiful and forbearing wife Nancy who provided the necessary domestic tranquility. Her vivacious personality shed sunlight into the darkest days of winter of which there are far too many in Ithaca, an otherwise wonderful place to live, and whose culinary talents make every dinner something to look forward to after a long day's work.

Introduction

This book asserts that the prevailing wisdom guiding health policy thinking is rooted in historical convictions and circumstances that have been overtaken by changes in social and economic development. Important changes in population structure and the global economy, compounded by costly advances in medical innovation and insatiable public demands for health care, underlie a need to re-examine and revise old beliefs and attitudes hampering meaningful health reform. This is apparent in the unsustainability of present rates of health spending and the many deficiencies in the way health care is structured and delivered. The necessity for a new health policy paradigm in which pragmatism counts for more than ideology comprises a unifying theme.

In addition to reassessing how to achieve affordable universal health coverage in the wake of alarming growth in the size of the uninsured population, policy makers need to reconsider the objective of private health insurance and the rights and responsibilities of individuals in matters of health maintenance and the payment of health services. While necessary, universal coverage alone is insufficient. Absent complementary structural improvements, spending will continue rising uncontrollably.

In the context of current health policy deliberations, universal coverage builds on coverage provided by employers and government programs. It requires that individuals not covered by other means purchase insurance coverage on their own. To ease the financial burden of doing so, government assistance is provided to low- and middle-income households on a sliding scale basis. Failure to comply is subject to financial penalties. In these respects the program closely follows a mandatory coverage model first introduced in the state of Massachusetts.

Despite past improvements health care remains surprisingly antiquated. It retains many of the elements of an earlier cottage industry period that are strikingly at odds with advanced managerial and corporate practices for attaining productivity and quality improvements. Obstinate resistance to modernization encountered in health care is circumscribed by a historically powerful medical culture that is slowly yielding to the imperatives of contemporary demands and expectations.

Progress in dealing with issues now at the forefront of health policy suffers moreover from the polarizing effects of doctrinaire polemics that belie the complexities involved and obscure the long-term financial ramifications of popular solutions. Practicality and pragmatism are advanced as an alternative to ideological panaceas in interest of promoting a more realistic mindset for dealing with today's health care dilemmas.

The organization of the book is built on the following premises:

• Health care is, paradoxically, one on the largest and most backward sectors of the economy.

• Strategies for universal health coverage fully reliant on government and employer financing are unrealistic.

• Health insurance will undergo radical change.

• National health insurance is an idea whose time has passed.

• Life style and illness pattern changes necessitate a reconsideration of individual responsibility for wellness and health maintenance.

• Consumer-driven health care is an idea whose time has arrived.

• Practical necessity points to a continuing and expanded role for market forces in health care.

• The complexities of today's health policy issues transcend ideological solutions.

The book consists of six chapters. Chapter 1 provides a standard overview of the health sector's economic size and significance, together with major structural flaws that underlie shortcomings in efficiency and quality controls and contribute to high rates of spending. Among the structural shortcomings considered are underinvestment in primary care, overspending on high-technology medicine, misaligned third-party financing incentives, pervasiveness of fraud and abuse, resistance to the adoption of information technology, and cottage industry legacy features that contribute to the fragmentation of services and lack of accountability on the part of the medical profession. Briefly stated, it argues that health care cost too much and produces too little. Passage of universal coverage, while essential, is insufficient. Without corollary reforms in the efficiency and quality, however, health spending will continue to grow at unsustainable levels.

Chapter 2 describes the politics of health reform in terms of the influence of special interests and the inescapability of compromise. Health care comprises almost 17 percent of a giant-sized national economy. It is characterized by unmatched complexity and composed of powerful interest groups with a long history of bending change to their advantage. With this in mind, the enormity of the task becomes staggering. Following a review of the special interests that health reform must accommodate if it is to succeed, the legacy of a deeply conservative health care culture is presented as another impediment to overcome. The tradition of medicine as a self-regulating profession and the functional imperatives for clinical autonomy are regarded as major reasons behind the slow progress in efficiency and quality improvements and why management is viewed as the enemy of good patient care. Suspicions against profit making in health care and the principle that individuals have a right to free health care as embodied in the ideology of national health insurance are reviewed together with the classic arguments justifying the exclusion of health care from the normal rules of market competition.

The role of powerful health culture values is examined more closely in chapter 3 in terms of society's inability to confront the hard qualitative and quantitative trade-offs inherent in the disproportionate health resources expended on the elderly and the physically and mentally impaired newborn, and the difficulty policy makers confront in attempting to reconcile belief in the right of individuals to universal comprehensive free health care with the constraints on public and employer financing. This discussion leads to an examination of the underlying reasons why the momentum for health spending is so resistant to control. The prime sources of inflationary spending are attributed to the contribution of third-party financing that inadvertently sustains the popular but erroneous idea that health care is a free good and the paternalistic feature of the physician–patient relationship that fosters dependency at the expense of consumer enfranchisement and solidifies mutually serving interests opposed to the imposition of modern managerial methods for efficiency and quality improvement.

Contrary to the prevailing wisdom, the uninsured are revealed as not constituting a financially disadvantaged homogeneous group. When disaggregated, a significant number of them chose to remain uninsured and numerous others would be able to purchase private coverage if assisted with sliding scale public subsidies, leaving a much smaller number totally reliant on public financing.

The contribution of market forces to alleviating the strains on public financing is further appraised in the context of their applicability to the utilization of routine health care needs and discretionary health services consumption, and this reveals that as much as 30 percent of health spending, contrary to popular belief, fits the definition of a consumer good. Reconnecting individuals to the economic consequences of their health care choices is presented as a practical means for slowing inflationary increases in health spending. The constructive role that market competition can perform in circumventing opposition to health reform from entrenched interests who are able to employ political influence to their advantage is presented as a hidden but important benefit of market competition.

Chapter 4 focuses on the ramifications of new demographic and economic realities that are redefining the role of government and employers. The message it contains is twofold. National health insurance orthodoxy will have to be rethought to accommodate the unhappy fact that the federal government has already promised more in entitlement benefits than it can deliver without substantially altering the terms of its implied contract with the American public, and the cost to employers of providing first dollar coverage to their employees is fast reaching a prohibitive level. This position, however, does not detract from the imperative for universal health coverage. Rather, it signals the need for greater creativity and practicality in meeting this goal.

Pursuit of national health insurance or single-payer coverage is presented as a utopian ideal that is divorced from contemporary realities. New economic and demographic realities point to a need to reconsider the degree to which insurance ought to shield individuals from health care costs. Increased individual responsibility, scaled to ability to pay, is regarded as requisite to devising a program of universal coverage that is fiscally responsible. In this context, requiring the uninsured to purchase health insurance along with the provision of sliding scale public subsidies to persons in financial need is the most practical means for assuring universal coverage. Financial exigencies for greater budgetary predictability and disciplined spending within the federal government foretell continued experimentation with managed care and a growing interest in the application of vouchers in Medicare and other government health programs—also that rejection of multi-tiered health care in which care is provided independently of income and wealth distinctions is unrealistic. The imperatives for greater fiscal responsibility also foretell the need for government to face up to the magnitude of the Social Security and Medicare financial crisis and to abandon the accounting chicanery of pay-as-you-go financing in favor of more prudent arrangements that require making actual deposits in the programs' trust funds.

In light of the aging of the labor force and growth in the size of the retiree population, on the one hand, and the emergence of global trade in which profits and survival are imperiled by high labor cost, on the other, this chapter concludes that employers are unlikely to remain the nation's main source of health insurance coverage. The economic pressures they encounter point to a much diminished role. The trend among small-sized firms to disengage totally from the provision of health benefits will not diminish, whereas large firms encumbered with high legacy costs will continue to pursue means for offloading retiree health coverage to others. In addition to current initiatives for shifting health cost increases to employees, firms continuing health insurance coverage predictably will focus more on providing protection against major medical expenses rather than first-dollar coverage. Whatever assistance is provided to employees for meeting the cost of routine health care needs will be in the form of health saving accounts. In the interest of better budgetary control, employers will seek to follow the precedent established with pension benefit programs and transform health care from a defined benefit to a defined contribution plan in which vouchers are an important component.

In the final analysis, discontinuation of employer coverage arguably is in the national interest inasmuch as it removes restrictions on job mobility and facilitates the more productive use of human capital. Toward this end, a change of ownership is anticipated whereby health insurance will be purchased by individuals rather than by employers or government, and tax benefits presently given to employers will be redirected to individuals. To preclude such socially dysfunctional practices as selective enrollment, denial of coverage for preexisting conditions, and discriminatory pricing based on age and health status, insurers will be compelled to enroll everyone who applies for coverage. A companion mandate requiring all individuals to possess basic health coverage will eliminate the justification for such undesirable practices, inasmuch as insurers are freed from adverse-selection risks that occur when uninsured individuals are able to put off enrolling until they either have or anticipate a need for coverage. Firms disproportionately impacted with more costly populations will be appropriately compensated from public funds, and in the interest of uniform national standards, regulation of the insurance industry will become a federal rather than remain a state government responsibility.

Chapter 5 illuminates and debunks a number of popular misconceptions that buttress the justification for a government takeover of health care. They include the assertion that national health insurance and its recently repackaged single-payer version offers the best way to cut health spending, the claim that more health spending is desirable for the reason that it results in improved health status and longevity, a belief in the superiority of centralized planning and control over the power of market forces in accomplishing public objectives, affirmation that investments in preventive medicine generate big savings, endorsement of single-payer coverage as the key to eliminating social and economic disparities in access to quality health care along with heath status and longevity, and the promulgation of the safety and efficacy of health care. The experience of other highly developed countries, England and Canada in particular, are cited in repudiating the soundness of many of these claims.

Because it increases and eases access to health care, the effect of national health insurance promotes rather than reduces spending, and in sustaining the notion that health care is a free good, it unwittingly feeds insatiable demands for spending growth that challenge the political will of government to counteract. This is a major reason why many advanced welfare state nations either have solicited or are considering private-sector partnerships.

The claim that heath spending is directly related to health status and longevity is questioned. While clearly applicable to poor and emerging economies, the relationship becomes ambivalent at higher levels of social and economic development where other factors intervene. In the case of infant mortality, factors like income distribution, education, and ethnic and religious composition account for more of the gains than does government health spending. As for spending on the elderly, the gains become problematic. From the standpoint of generating the national wealth required to pay for expanding retirement and other social welfare services, financial imperatives necessitate consumption–investment trade-offs and a shift in focus from the prolongation of life to health services that improve productivity.

Savings from preventive medicine moreover are criticized for being exaggerated due to the paradox of medicine that enables persons who otherwise would have died to survive but with a need for continuing care and to life-cycle stages where costly forms of chronic illness and disability become more prevalent. Preventive medicine, broadly defined, encompasses the benefits of early detection and management of chronic conditions as well as disease avoidance. For the most part, neither health screening nor disease management practices have been demonstrated to save money over the long run. More important, they often expose individuals to unnecessary treatment risks that result in doing far more harm than good.

Because of the Law of Inverse Need whereby the supply and quality of health resources flow disproportionately to privileged areas and because also of the effects of cultural differences in lifestyle behaviors and other factors, absolute health levels may improve but relative differences remain and often enlarge. The difficulty of eliminating health disparities is substantiated by the inability of the British National Health Service to do so despite the purported advantages of public financing and centralized planning and control.

The reputed benefits of centralized planning and control belie the vast complexities of health care that defy the analytic power of models devised by experts. Regulatory authority for its part is susceptible to capture by the very special interests it presumably controls. The complexity of health care is manifest furthermore in the difficulty of devising efficacy and effectiveness standards that account for the inherent ambiguities in clinical medicine and the cost and complexity of conducting clinical trials involving human subjects.

Contrary to its image for scientific excellence, the safety and efficacy of modern medicine is woefully inadequate. Due partly to an over reliance on paper records, medical error rates are shockingly high. Moreover medially questionable and/or unnecessary differences in the treatment of illness and its associated costs within and across geographic areas are rampant. Much of modern medical practice rests on standards other than conclusive scientific evidence because of the lack of systemic procedures.

Chapter 6 readdresses the reasons behind the need for a new health policy paradigm that is attuned to the realities of the new economy, an aging population, and the escalating costs attributable to medical innovation. These realities urge the acquiescence of ideology to pragmatism in the interest of harnessing the power of private interest for the attainment of otherwise unaffordable and unattainable social objectives. Based on the nature of health care issues and trends analyzed in preceding chapters, a number of conclusions appear evident: Employers will cease being the primary source of health insurance coverage. The federal government lacks the capacity to take on sole responsibility for financing new and costly entitlement programs. The idealized version of national health insurance, including its single-payer counterpart, is an idea whose time has passed. The equalitarian principles undergirding Medicare that prohibit differential treatment by income are fast eroding. Upper income beneficiaries will be required to contribute more and receive less. Full benefits will be paid only to those who truly need them; all others will be cut back. Cost containment strategies that fail to share efficiency savings with consumers are unlikely to succeed. Constraints on government and employer financing indicate that entirely free health care is unfeasible.

In conclusion, this book asserts that health policy has reached a turning point. The influence of ideology that has dominated past disputes over health reform is fading. Increasingly policy makers are defying popular orthodoxies and accommodating new realities. New realities compel a re-examination of underlying conventional assumptions and beliefs on how best to finance and deliver health care. For similar reasons liberal and conservative disputes that have deterred efforts to introduce modern managerial principles to correct inadequate efficiency and quality control practices are steadily being relegated to the margins in favor of more practical approaches.

Frustration over the stalemate in health reform attributable to the polarizing effects of ideologically driven solutions pushes decision makers to subordinate the ideal in favor of the practical. The visible trend toward a higher regard for pragmatism and practicality in the United States as well as abroad reflects the emergence of a more intellectually sober understanding of the inflationary ramifications of implementing idealized versions of universal free health care.

1   Health Policy: Then and Now

Health policy has undergone a profound transformation in the post–World War II period. Massive growth, both in size and significance, has propelled it to the forefront of national attention. This contrasts sharply with its former status as a distinct component of the national economy. The rate at which already large-sized outlays are now growing stirs concerns about whether the health sector is consuming too large a share of national income at a time when pressures are mounting to expand public spending to support a growing number of uninsured Americans. Political controversy over whether and how to deal with the uninsured problem is compounded by an accumulation of strains on the federal budget that questions whether it is prudent for government to add to the size of presently unfunded commitments to health care in order to make universal coverage possible. In the interest of avoiding wasteful spending, a consensus is emerging that a major expansion of public financing is not feasible unless measures are included for addressing serious shortcomings in the way health services are structured and delivered.

Reforming health care, however, poses a formidable challenge inasmuch as the health sector today is, paradoxically, one of the biggest and most antiquated components of the national economy. This paradox, as reflected in the gap between the technology of medicine and the way health services are organized and delivered, was recognized as far back as the mid-1940s. What is truly amazing is how little progress has occurred since then in introducing modern managerial principles for efficiency and quality assurance. This more than anything else speaks to the resiliency and obduracy of entrenched health care interests and the enormity of the political challenge confronting the current leadership for health reform (Berge 1958: 666–67).

While the subject of health reform has a long history expending back to the earliest of many failed attempts to enact national health insurance close to a century ago, the sense of urgency for comprehensive restructuring and modernization is quite recent. It is fueled by growing unease over the sustainability of present rates of growth in health spending, evidence that the nation does not compare favorably with other industrial nations in the value obtained from health spending, criticism that too much money is lavished on costly high-technology medical services to the neglect of less costly basic health care needs, the dysfunctionality of a system of financing that rewards waste and inefficiency, the difficulty of meeting modern efficiency and quality standards within an outdated health care infrastructure, and the counterproductive effects of overly legalistic means for holding health care providers accountable for substandard care. The urgency for reform spurred by these concerns is the subject of this chapter.

Growth of Health Spending

Prior to the mid-1960s the amount of national income going to health care was too small to arouse concern about how new program costs would affect the general economy. Rather than worry about the ramifications for economic growth and living standards of future generations, the priority centered instead on eliminating price and income barriers for low-income persons. Although, beginning in the Second World War, private health insurance coverage spread rapidly throughout the population, it failed, whether due to inability or unwillingness, to include the many elderly, indigent, and working poor. Medicare and Medicaid, enacted in 1965, were specifically designed to close this gap.

Making coverage available to persons most in need of health care but who could least afford it, the enactment of Medicare and Medicaid was driven by deep moral misgivings over the anomaly of needy persons being deprived of health care within a rich society. Moreover expanding affluence was popularly believed to have become a permanent economic fixture (Galbraith 1958). The sharp divide between persons with and without adequate income as well as access to health care was denounced as an affront to the nation's humanitarian standing by egalitarian-minded social reformers, all the more so because it was widely believed among progressive intellectuals that economists had acquired the knowledge to control fluctuations in the business cycle and manage prosperity. This, of course, soon proved to be highly exaggerated as the economy quickly resumed its normal pattern of swinging unpredictably between periods of boom and bust (Samuelson 2008).

Any residual belief in the power of government policy to control economic events evaporated with the enormous loss of wealth in 2008 caused by the second worst collapse of the economy since the Great Depression and was preceded by alarmingly large increases in private and public debt levels. In a dramatic shift from earlier decades, financial turmoil and uncertainty shapes today's policy deliberations on whether too much of the nation's wealth is being spent on health services.

In the economic and social circumstances of the 1960s, policy discussion centered more on the possibility that the nation was spending too little rather than too much on health care. Hospital and physician services were fairly inexpensive by current measures, since clinical medicine was still in its infancy. From the standpoint of having a large number of effective therapies, medicine was just entering the threshold of major breakthroughs and the treatments available were not as technologically intensive and costly as they are today (e.g., see NY Academy of Medicine 1958: 115–21; Cutler 2004: 1–9; Le Fanu 1999). Consequently the money required to broaden access to health care through voluntary health insurance and government programs was not an urgent concern. Passing national health insurance was seen more as a matter of political will.

Much of what was available to physicians at the time was still carried in an iconic little black bag. The increase in life expectancy prior to that time was due more to rising living standards and public health improvements in sanitation, food safety, and communicable disease control than advances in clinical medicine (Illich 1975; McKeown 1976; McKinlay 1980: 3–16).

Stoked initially by the vast infusion of government funds following enactment of Medicare and Medicaid, and subsequent improvements in clinical medicine, the amount of health spending as a portion of the gross domestic product (GDP) measure jumped from 5 percent in the early postwar years to a current level of 17 percent. Because of a historic pattern in which health care is expected to continue growing two to three times faster than the general economy, it is projected, barring corrective action, to account for about 20 percent or more of GDP by 2015 (National Coalition on Health Care 2009; US Department of Health and Human Services 2007). Whether such growth is sustainable and in the national interest is problematic. Apart from any purported benefits, spending of such magnitude stirs fears that it is or soon will crowd out expenditures for other important priorities (Congressional Budget Office 2008). However, slowing the pace of increase in spending and reforming health care is easier said than done.

In addition to issues of complexity and the political difficulty of overcoming a formidable array of interest groups vested in the status quo, health spending, ironically, acquires a measure of immunity from criticism in severe economic downturns. Because health care is one of the few recession proof areas and source of new jobs in periods of high unemployment, policies aimed at reducing spending are considered counterproductive. Health care today is a powerful machine capable of both creating and sustaining jobs. It is the nation's biggest industry and forecast to create more jobs over the next decade than all other industries combined, thus making a virtue out of otherwise doubtful spending. Localities with a declining economic base and unemployment are unlikely to tamper with health care employment and spending. It is viewed as a critical source of income and a shelter against further job loss and economic decline.

Health Spending Value

Other industrialized countries spend less and get more for their money than does the United States. In national income terms (GDP), the United States outspends the next highest spender by three percentage points. The per capita spread is higher yet, at least 24 percent, more than the next biggest spenders and 90 percent or more than other countries that can be considered economic competitors (Organization for Economic Cooperation and Development 2006). Yet the results are mediocre. Although other factors play a role, these differences in national spending reflect, in large part, how medical innovation is absorbed in the delivery of health services.

The national pride stirred by the international acclaim enjoyed by the National Institutes of Health and top medical centers is magnified by the envy foreigners' often display over the abundance of high-technology services in the United States and the few restrictions on their use. Indeed the prominence given to high-technology medicine underlies the outpouring of boastful pronouncements proclaiming the preeminence of American medicine; the affirmation of which is derived from the many rich and famous foreigners who, when confronted with life-threatening medical conditions, opt for US hospitals and physicians. This image, however, belies some glaring deficiencies. (For an overview of how the

United States differs from other countries where health services are better organized, see Reid 2009.)

When compared to other countries that spend far less, the United States ranks poorly in a number of basic health measures as infant mortality, child well-being, life expectancy, and mortality rates for cancer and cardiovascular diseases. It is the only highly developed country that fails to provide universal health coverage for its citizens (Anderson and Frogner 2008; United Health Foundation 2008). Much of the blame for this is attributable to the nation's predilection for prestigious, but costly, high-technology medicine, on the one hand, and a corresponding neglect of unglamorous low-technology health services for routine medical and preventative services, on the other.

Preoccupation with High Technology

Leadership in medical technology is a defining feature of US health care and helps explain why spending surpasses levels found in other industrial nations. Unlike the United States, other countries concentrate first on developing and maintaining a strong base of inexpensive primary care services essential to disease prevention and health maintenance before investing heavily in technologically intensive patient care. Economic necessity, if not enlightened decision-making, leads countries less wealthy than the United States to carefully scrutinize the cost-effectiveness as well as safety and efficacy of new technologies and to limit their availability to all but the most advanced and specialized medical centers. This form of rationing, however, is anathema in the United States where the idea of having to wait for elective procedures and other treatments is highly unpopular. Therefore much less differentiation in the services is found in community hospitals and big medical centers than in most countries, where a hierarchical distribution of services based and their cost and complexity is the rule. The types of diagnostic technologies found in physicians' offices follows a similar pattern (Garber and Skinner 2008).

In addition to scoring poorly in international comparisons of basic health indexes, this fascination with high technology is mirrored in differences in the supply of generalist physicians to medical specialists. Countries that spend less and appear to get a better return on their money have a higher ratio of primary care practitioners to specialists, whereas specialists dominate the US medical scene, to a degree that having too few primary care practitioners is a persistent problem. In other developed countries between 50 to 75 percent of physicians are in primary care whereas in the United States only 35 percent are in primary care (Starfield 2000).

Differences in prestige combined with income differentials put primary care practitioners at a disadvantage and discourage medical students from entering the field. Reimbursement and compensation practices heavily favor specialists. Physician payment in the Medicare program continues to be fee for service, although it was redesigned in the early 1990s to entice more physicians into choosing primary care as a career by decreasing the disparity in income with surgical specialties. While an admirable objective, the remaining gap has been too large to significantly alter shortages in the supply of primary care physicians (Feldstein 2007).

The definition of primary care further illuminates differences in reliance on costly technologies. In lower spending countries primary care is provided exclusively by general practitioners, a type of practice that no longer exists in the United States. Primary care consists instead of a several medical specialties—family medicine, general internal medicine, and pediatrics. General practitioners not only cost less to educate but having them provide for most individual and family routine health needs does much to contain supply-induced demand effects on health spending that flows from physicians' motivation—whether self-esteem, prestige, or income considerations—to do what they have been trained to do. Reliance on general practitioners for meeting basic individual and family health needs curbs such tendencies because, unlike US primary care practitioners, they typically lack hospital privileges and direct access to expensive diagnostic tools and laboratory testing (Stephen 1979).

Disproportionate spending on high-technology medicine also contributes to the large number of Americans without health insurance. It stresses the financing of job-connected coverage, whereby most insurance is paid by employers, and puts insurance beyond the reach of the self-employed and unemployed who must pay for health insurance on their own. Individuals working for firms not offering insurance comprise, together with their dependents, the single largest group among the uninsured (Center for Medicare and Medicaid Services 2007).

In cases where employees are offered coverage, the rejection rate among low-income workers is growing commensurate with the out-of-pocket burden created as employers increasingly shift all or part of higher insurance costs to them. Business- and industry-sponsored efforts over the past several decades to slow growth in insurance premium prices have focused on initiatives aimed at changing inflationary hospital and physician practices. However, apart from temporary gains, they have not been able to arrest the momentum for higher spending.

Cutbacks in employment benefits, coupled with a steep rise in jobless numbers during periods of economic decline, test the capacity of public and voluntary social service agencies to meet increased household demands for assistance. Meanwhile the stress induced by unemployment and loss of income is correlated with an increase in mortality and the onset of serious physical and mental health problems (Catalano 2009: 749–51; Brenner 1987, 1997). The social and economic fallout highlights the disadvantage of tying health insurance coverage to employment status and amplifies appeals for national health insurance—recently reincarnated as single-payer coverage (Pear 2008: 30n; Sack 2008).

Many factors contribute to health care spending and cost—such as population increase and aging, inflation, scope of insurance coverage and consumer purchasing power, and supplier-induced demand—but medical innovation clearly is the most important, accounting for over half of spending increases (Newhouse 1992). Concerns about the quality of care problems, inefficiency, and low productivity are rooted in the pervasiveness of high technology. This is partly reflected in the rate at which highly specialized procedures are done.

Among highly developed countries the United States is the undisputed leader in the number of coronary bypass, coronary angioplasty, and kidney transplant procedures performed per 100,000 persons. Moreover it has twice as many CT scanners and three times as many MRI machines per capita as found on average in other highly developed countries (Peterson and Burton 2007). An abundance of intensive neonatal resources provides another example. The United States has 3.3 intensive care beds per 10,000 live births versus 2.6 for Australia and Canada, and 0.67 for the United Kingdom (Thompson, Goodman, and Little 2002).

Ironically, high-technology medicine is a source of patient harm whenever, as often occurs in the United States, physicians expose patients to medical risks by overprescribing diagnostic imaging that emit potentially harmful radiation and laboratory tests that additionally can falsely point to the need for medical and surgical treatments, or whenever physicians perform an insufficient number of complex procedures required to maintain skill levels for favorable outcomes, such as heart bypass surgery. Failure to employ high-technology services to full capacity moreover is economically wasteful. It results in higher unit costs and questionable duplication of services (e.g., see Millenson 1997; Kling 2006). Minimizing such problems is, of course, a principal benefit from controlling the diffusion of costly technologies and organizing health services within a hierarchy of ascending complexity. Technological proliferation in the United States is a reflection of the abundance of money available for health care as well as ineffectual diffusion controls and the method of paying for health care.

Perverse Effects of Health Financing

The method of payment for hospitals and physicians also has a big impact on health spending. The method of reimbursement followed in the United States is highly inflationary. It represents an extension of an earlier historic practice in which health providers set their own fees and patients were solely responsible for payment. Pricing was restrained by the limited capacity of household incomes and the intimacy of doctor–patient relationships. This worked as long as health care remained inexpensive and household were able to pay privately.

The interposition of third parties and rise of well-financed insurance companies in the aftermath of the Great Depression had a dramatic opposite effect. It created the perception that health care had become a free good, an illusion springing from the World War II public policy decision granting employers tax incentives to become the primary provider of health insurance to workers and their families. This dramatically reduced the need for out-of-pocket payments since, at the time, it was normal for employers to pay the full premiums and first-dollar coverage was the norm. This free-good illusion, when combined with the uninterrupted freedom of hospitals and physicians to set their own fees, established a dynamic for excess spending that, with few interruptions, has continued to the present (Cannon and Tanner 2005: 45–59).

Among the insured, medical bills ceased being a problem, while hospitals and physicians were induced to overproduce services because their income varied not only by the fees they charged but also by the volume of procedures performed. Reimbursement was open ended, and providers retained wide latitude in what they charged. Payments were unquestioned, thereby creating an additional incentive to practice with little if any regard for economy. Submitting services to any form of cost–benefit analysis was unimaginable in this free-good heyday. Nor was there any compulsion for self-restraint.

Health providers did not lose control over pricing until the early 1980s when the federal government sought to limit Medicare spending by imposing a system of administered diagnostic-specific prices on hospitals. This development, together with growth in managed care enrollments, gave third-party purchasers such as Medicare and private insurers a stronger voice in negotiating lower fees. Despite provider's loss of pricing powers, the incentive to overproduce has continued because providers simply expand volume to compensate for any price reductions.

Health providers have also learned to manipulate the Medicare and related payment systems by focusing on high–profit margin diagnoses, among which cardiac surgery is a favorite selection. Creative billing practices in which procedures are broken down into the largest possible number of components and billed separately along with the selection of more severe and complex diagnostic codes, the justification of which are open to subjective differences of expert opinion, comprise yet other ways hospitals and physicians evade third-party price controls (Cannon and Tanner 2005: 49–51).

Unfortunately, to this day providers are paid regardless of the quality of their care. Quality care and poor care are reimbursed equally. Providers benefit from their mistakes. Ironically, they are paid twice for treating the same condition, such as hospital readmissions, thereby creating a disincentive to improve treatment standards. This is poised to change, however. Momentum is building for performance-based compensation. Medicare has launched a policy of denying payments to hospitals for certain avoidable medical errors, and private insurers are starting to move in a similar direction. By and large, however, it remains a serious problem (Fuhrmans 2008).

It is unrealistic to expect that the tendency of physicians to overproduce health services can be corrected by paying them differently (Tulchinsky and Varavikova 2009: 426). Independent of how compensated, it is difficult for physicians to refrain from doing what they have been trained to do. Roughly 75 percent of all health spending is said to be the result of decisions made by physicians on behalf of patients. Recognition that each medical school graduate going into patient care invariably makes diagnostic and treatment decisions that result in costly expenditures is why many countries seek to control the supply of physicians by capping medical school admissions and limiting entry into medical specialties (Garber and Skinner 2008). However, this sort of governmental intervention remains too unpopular to implement in the United States because of the value placed on freedom of choice and individualism.

In place of a uniform national health workforce policy, physician supply decisions mainly are determined by the needs of medical schools and teaching hospitals along with a private advisory body on graduate medical education that speaks on behalf of a collection of medical interest groups in overseeing residency training. The only direct control exercised by the federal government is on the inflow of foreign physicians who are allowed to practice in the country.

The US government exercises an indirect influence on medical education through the imposition of limits on the payments it makes to teaching hospitals for the training of medical residents through the Medicare program. However, teaching institutions remain free to find their own sources of money to expand the number of residencies they offer. Thus the government's influence is limited to discouraging teaching hospitals from increasing the number of residency positions (Iglehart 2008; Croasdale 2006).

The cost problems spawned by provider reimbursement are made worse by the multiplicity of third parties. It is not unusual for physicians to contract with as many as twenty insurance companies, each of which has different reimbursement and reporting criteria (Practice Management Resources Medical Group Management Association 2004). The resulting red tape and paper work are a drag on efficiency and contribute to high administrative expenses. The clerical and related compliance costs of dealing with multiple insurance companies contribute substantially to the overhead cost of maintaining a private medical practice, typically around 60 percent of gross revenues.

It is estimated that roughly 20 percent of insurance firms' outlays for hospital and physician services go to billing- and insurance-related functions (Kahn et al. 2005). Indeed the extra health care costs incurred from working with so many different insurers is a major argument in favor of going to a single-payer system. For all practical purposes, single-payer health care is a synonym for national health insurance, inasmuch as the government pays for care that is universal and comprehensive, while ownership and management of physician and hospital services remains in private hands. Single pay is largely based on the Canadian health care model. Although retaining fee-for-service reimbursement, the Canadian government resorts to controls over capital expenditures and the supply of physicians and health facilities in order to maintain disciplined spending. In addition access to elective procedures is rationed through means of waiting lists (Garber and Skinner 2008).

Proponent of single pay see no social benefit from having multiple insurers, particularly in light of the associated administrative cost that amounts to nearly one-fourth of all health spending (Woolhandler, Himmelstein, and Lewontin 2003). Marketing expenses and payments to investors and executive salaries absorb approximately 20 percent of the premium dollar in for-profit plans. The amount for not-for-profit plans is roughly 10 percent. They do not have shareholders to deal with and generally pay executives less, but nevertheless have marketing and sales costs. Medicare in comparison is far more efficient. Spared market place expenses and benefiting from economies of scale, it spends only around 2 to 3 percent for administration and overhead (Matthews 2006). This suggests to single-payer supporters the possibility of generating from $100 to$200 billion in efficiency savings, a sum they believe is sufficient to meet the cost of granting universal coverage to the uninsured population and upgrade coverage for underinsured persons (Himmelstein and Woolhandler 2003).

Coping with the public–private mix of third parties adds to the aggravations and cost of health care delivery. Single-payer health care is no panacea, however. Government funded programs are notorious for the volume of ill-defined regulations and cumbersome reimbursement practices, many examples of which are found in Medicare and Medicaid (Aaron 2003). Especially troubling to medical interests is the latest attempt by the federal government to control what it spends yearly on physician services in the Medicare program by eliminating or curtailing cost of living increases to physicians whenever total spending grows faster than the general economy—an action taken in the belief that it had been overly generous in paying physicians in the past.

Because the formula is highly complicated and confusing, and subject to political grandstanding by members of Congress, physicians now perceive their income to be under constant threat. Income anxiety, together with difficulties involved in billing and claims processing, is a source of irritation that, if unattended, may lead physicians to withdraw from Medicare participation and, in so doing, make it more difficult for the elderly to access health care (Feldstein 2007: 125–38).

Hospitals too are subjected to similar stress from Medicare reporting requirements and shortsighted payment formula changes, which then push them to skirt the outer edges of ethical behavior in order to offset money-losing services. In addition to the ramifications for quality cited earlier, hospitals have resorted to the cost-shifting practice of charging private insurers more in order to compensate for cutbacks in government payments (Congressional Budget Office 2008). The added cost of doing business, of course, eventually causes employers to shift cost increases to their employees, feeding in turn a downward spiral toward an inability to afford health care.

Medicaid, if anything, is an even worse example of bureaucratic complexity and poor payment history. Because of the role of state governments, Medicaid is an amalgam of 50 separate programs in which eligibility criteria, reporting rules, and provider reimbursement widely vary. What these two programs have in common is a reputation for being bad payers. They share a tendency to pay health providers far below their operating costs and to delay what payments they approve far beyond normal business standards. Medicare and Medicaid underpayment of hospitals and physicians results in a hidden tax amounting to nearly $90 billion that is shifted to private insurers and ultimately to employers and consumers in the form of higher premiums, amounting to roughly $1,500 or more than 10 percent of the cost for a family of four. For Medicare, hospitals receive payment of only 91 cents for every dollar they spend in caring for Medicare patients. For Medicaid, hospitals receive only 88 cents for every dollar they spend in caring for Medicaid patients. Physicians fare worse. Medicare pays them 89 percent of their usual fee whereas Medicaid pays only 60 percent of their usual fee. The result is that private payers pay 14 percent more on average (Fox and Pickering 2008). Medicaid underpayment only compounds the problems the poor have in getting health care. In 2003, for example, only 40 percent of physicians accepted all new Medicaid patients and the percentage of physicians not accepting any new Medicaid patients was around 30 percent (Cannon and Tanner 2005: 101–102).

Compared with the federal government, the states have less flexibility in funding health programs, since they are legally compelled to balance their budgets. They also have a smaller tax base and lack the power to print money. Loss of revenues during economic downturns and higher unemployment therefore affects them more directly, and budgetary crisis occur more frequently. When trimming spending to balance budgets to offset revenue shortfalls, state officials invariably focus on Medicaid as a source of savings, since it is one of the biggest and fastest growing components of state government operating expenditures. Medicaid now accounts for more than one-fifth of total state expenditures, second only to elementary and secondary education (National Association of State Budget Officers 2002).

Despite federal matching contributions ranging from 50 to 80 percent, the states have trouble meeting their share of Medicaid spending during recessionary times. The reason is that Medicaid rolls inconveniently rise just as the economy weakens and tax revenues fall. If forced with a choice of how to economize in social safety net programs when confronted with rising unemployment and poverty rates, cutting payments to health providers most often emerges as the least damaging in a mixture of undesirable options. The negative spillover effects of underpaying health providers go beyond discouraging physician participation to include undesirable hospital cost-shifting practices and, more regrettably, enticements for fraud and abuse that are abetted by weak financial oversight of billings submitted by health care providers. The same applies to Medicare.

Fraud and Abuse

While an impressive amount, the nearly $2 billion in fines and settlements collected by the federal government in 2007, practically speaking, understates the extent of this Medicare and Medicaid problem by an unknown but large amount; fraud and abuse by their very nature are unknown until detected (Aronivitz 2005). Since systematic effort to crack down on the problem began in 1997, over $11 billion has been restored to the Medicare Trust Fund (US Department of Health and Human Services and US Department of Justice 2008). It is safe to conclude from this that fraud and abuse is pervasive in the health sector. Most such estimates range from a low of 3 percent to as much as 10 percent of all spending (National Health Care Anti-Fraud Association 2009; FBI 2007). A major reason why better information is lacking is that fraud detection is not a high priority. Unlike private insurers, Medicare and Medicaid automatically pay all submitted bills containing a valid claims number. In comparison, private insurers have higher administrative costs, partly because they routinely screen for waste and fraud in addition to spending on programs aimed at building networks of trustworthy health care providers. Underinvestment in administrative overhead in Medicare and Medicaid thus creates an invitation to steal. According to Malcom Sparrow, a Harvard professor of public management who has examined the scope of the problem, as much as 20 to 30 percent of federal health spending is consumed by fraud. As a share of Medicare spending, this may amount to $85 billion a year (Sparrow 2009).

Cottage Industry Features

Health sector backwardness is especially obvious in the manner in which health care is delivered. A major problem is it that it is essentially a high-tech cottage industry. Although considerable consolidation has occurred since the 1990s when hospitals and physicians began to counter the pricing power acquired by insurance firms by merging into larger entities, health care retains many of the features characteristic of a cottage industry. It still has too many small-sized providers to capitalize on today's sophisticated managerial and technological means for efficiency improvement and quality control (McKinsey and Company 2008). Most providers, for example, have too small a presence in the marketplace to obtain the price discounts suppliers of health products grant to larger buyers (Reinhardt, Hussey, and Anderson 2004).

Nearly 50 percent of all hospitals have fewer than 100 beds, notwithstanding a trend, beginning in the mid-1980s, marking the closure of small hospitals, particularly in rural areas. Fewer than 20 percent have 300 or more beds (US Department of Health and Human Services 2006). Notwithstanding around 700 mergers between 1996 and 2000, insufficient hospital scale remains a problem (Porter and Teisberg 2004). Too many small facilities is an even bigger problem in the long-term care area, where evidence of substandard care is commonplace due to difficulties in staff hiring and retention and fragile financing (US Department of Health and Human Services 2006; Consumers Union 2003).

Similar insufficiency of scale problems characterizes the organization of physician services. Over 40 percent of physicians practice in groups with fewer than six colleagues while one-fourth of all physicians practice solo (Practice Management Resources Medical Group Management Association 2005). Fewer than 13 percent of small-sized medical groups are invested in electronic records (Miller and Sim 2004).

Fragmentation, and the barrier it poses to the coordination of patient care, is another outdated feature. Health care in its present configuration is better geared to acute disease patterns of yesteryear than the chronic degenerative disorders that are a feature of modern living and aging societies. Unlike acute communicable conditions that occur suddenly without the presence of other complicating conditions, and can be dealt with by a single physician, chronic disorders take years before they become obvious. Treatment is complicated because of the presence of additional health problems that are best dealt with by a team approach involving a number of different medical specialties together with other health personnel (Mechanic 2006: 8–11).

In countries where services are better structured, coordination is the function of a medical generalist—namely general practitioners—whom patients must first consult in nonemergency situations before they are permitted to see a specialist. In the United States, individuals are free, with the exception of some managed care plans, to consult any physician they prefer so that no one is formally in charge of coordinating their care. Disease prevention and health maintenance are neglected in the process, and treatment outcomes suffer therefore because of a lack of systematic follow-up. Even in those instances where patients are enrolled in health plans featuring coordinated care, investments in prevention and wellness programs are impeded because of frequent turnover among enrollees who leave the plan annually, either on their own or because their employer contracts with another health plan. Adoption of information technology is another problem. Unlike most industries that have escaped from reliance on paper, the health sector is a massive communications quagmire entangled in paper. Some 90 percent of physicians and two-thirds of hospitals continue to record patient data on paper, and among those who use digital data, there is frequently an inability to exchange information with outside parties, which reintroduces the need for paper (Weisman 2008). More important, dependence on paper impedes good follow-up when patients move on to other health care providers.

Digital interconnectedness making it possible for patient's medical information to be quickly transmitted from one provider to another is long overdue. Although medical error rates decline and efficiency improves when hospitals and physicians' offices go digital, the benefits remain localized if, as is the case presently, the information technology used differs between and among providers. Linkage within a shared standardized information system is essential to overcoming the inefficiencies inherent in the existing archaic and chaotic array of health services, inasmuch as a uniform electronic highway permits health care to function as a system where previously there was none (Merritt 2007). Achieving such integration is consequently a top priority within the information-system research community.

Litigious Impairment of Quality Improvement

Another facet that differentiates US health care from other countries is the legal environment within which care is provided and the agitation clouding deliberations on whether, by holding health providers accountable for their actions, it functions to support or deter quality patient care. Health providers, for the most part, agree that resolving quality of care disputes by litigation in which decisions are made by medically uninformed jurors has spiraled out of control because of the magnitude of monetary awards; it needs to be replaced by something better. The medical community conveys considerable stress over having to deal with such medical malpractice issues as the cost and availability of liability insurance, and also the proclivity of the courts to grant large monetary awards to plaintiffs. Perceived susceptibility to baseless claims and legal extortion that pressures health providers to settle out of court rather than endure high legal fees and unpredictable jury findings provokes anger and feelings of helplessness, along with a visceral dislike of tort lawyers.

Sensational accounts abound about how the cost of insurance coverage, for example, amounts of $75,000 to $100,000 for physicians in high-risk specialties like obstetrics and surgery impel physicians to retreat to a lower risk specialty or relocate to another state having lower insurance costs and a less threatening legal climate, thereby making it harder for patients to get health care. Malpractice insurance regulation is a state function and premium charges, accordingly, vary considerably. In order to slow physician flight, all but fifteen states have placed limits on medical malpractice awards. (For an example of press coverage, see Nixon 2008.)

However, not everyone agrees on the existence of a malpractice insurance crisis. Skeptics allege talk of crisis is overblown in order to insulate health care providers from being held accountable for their mistakes in causing injury and harm to patients and to bail out insurance firms by putting a cap on claims payments. They submit that price hikes in premiums are due less to litigation costs than to insurance firms having to raise rates for earlier underpricing strategies aimed at grabbing market share. In support of this argument is cited evidence that as few as one percent of medical mistakes result in a malpractice claim. Health providers' complaints of having to practice costly defensive medicine are dismissed as self-serving, inasmuch as fee-for-service reimbursement rewards them for every diagnostic test they order. Supporters of malpractice litigation hold that given the unavailability of an alternative, it is the only way hospitals and physicians can be held accountable for errors and outright malpractice. (See collection of news stories at MakeThemAccountable 2008.)

Such exchanges of the shortcomings and benefits of malpractice litigation miss the mark. They distract attention from the larger issue of how quality of care can be improved through better reporting of medical errors. A poorly admitted consequence of the litigation of quality control is the role that negative sanctions play in keeping health providers from learning from their mistakes. Abhorrence of the possible financial burden of litigation and harm to professional reputation is accentuated by the dread of having to endure the tedium of lengthy trial proceedings. It feeds evasion and denial. In order to flourish, quality control and opportunity for continuous improvement require a supportive atmosphere in which inadvertent mistakes serve as important learning tools. Other industries practice this routinely. That health care does not is no longer acceptable.

Quality Control Deficiencies

Until recently a lack of transparency shielded health care from public scrutiny. But the situation has changed now that it is no longer assumed, as it was historically, that medicine is just too complicated to be understood by ordinary citizens. A cascade of statistics depicting the poor state of quality control reveals what was previously hidden. Hospitals are dangerous to one's health! According to a report compiled by the National Institute of Medicine, up to 100,000 people die there annually as the result of medical mistakes and the chance of being injured in a hospital increase about 6 percent for each day of stay (Institute of Medicine 2000). If anything, the dangers are much larger than indicated because of the reluctance of hospitals to keep detailed records that can be used against them in malpractice suits. Taking all sources into account, it is believed that medical errors are the third leading cause of death in the United States (Starfield 2000). In addition to the pain and suffering involved, medical errors drive up the cost of health care by necessitating additional medical treatment and extending hospital stays. A study of eighteen types of preventable injuries, including infections, concluded that the extra charges per case totaled close to $60,000 (Zhan, Chunliu, and Miller 2003).

Notwithstanding recent year gains, more is needed to improve transparency, both with respect to error reporting and making information available in user-friendly ways so that individuals can make informed decisions in choosing hospitals and physicians. This alone, however, while necessary is insufficient. Better use is required of information age technologies for the implementation of quality control systems that eliminate hard to read handwritten orders and enable systematic checks for minimizing human error during all phases of patient care. Early signs of progress occurring within specific health care organizations are encouraging. Yet the larger challenge of interconnecting providers and patients with one another to form a seamless delivery system for expediting the flow of financial and health information to enable better-coordinated patient care at lower costs remains an important unmet national priority. Recently enacted federal legislation addresses this issue. The 2009 American Recovery and Reinvestment Act (ARRA) was passed to accelerate the adoption of information technology through financial incentives and penalties aimed at getting physicians and hospitals to adopt and use electronic records. The ARRA contains provisions also for laying the groundwork for uniform standards and nationwide interconnectedness However, the tangible benefits of such investment will not be seen for over a decade or more. (Blumenthal 2009).

Clearly, much remains to be done if the United States is to rightfully claim the title of having the world's best health care. Compared to other economically advanced countries, US health care badly lags behind in the number of people it reaches and in the quality of care it provides. Changing this situation is the paramount goal of health reform.

2 Resistance to Change

If the past is any indication of what can be expected, health reform is a goal more easily discussed than accomplished. Failed attempts to enact national health insurance extend back nearly a century and testify to the power of interests arrayed in support of the status quo (Anderson 1958: 621–28). Today's proposal goes far beyond universal coverage to encompass an ambitious overhaul of the coverage and deliverance of health care. What is contemplated is nothing less than the modernization of a badly antiquated health care structure. Given the scope and complexity of this undertaking, the confidence exhibited by reform proponents appears to be overly optimistic. This is not to say that progress is unattainable so much as to suggest that headway, as in the past, will be strongly contested and that any gains are apt to be incremental rather than sweeping in nature.

Year after year detailed plans for changing health care have been put forward amid great optimism only to ultimately collapse when countered by the objections of special interest groups (Daschle 2008). This time, however, the politics of reform may have reached a favorable tipping point due, paradoxically, to the economic distress gripping the nation. Compulsions for immediate action accompanying a crisis can help, if skillfully exploited, stifle opposition and avert momentum-robbing debate and compromises. Within the prevailing crisis-laden psychological climate, fed by plunging family incomes and middle-class anxiety over the stability of employment-based health coverage and job security, the circumstances appear especially auspicious for marshaling public support and assembling winning political coalitions (Helrman et al. 2009).

In the past, national health insurance lacked political traction because the uninsured and poor were too few in numbers to make a political difference. Middle-class indifference stemming from economic comfort tended to marginalize the significance of the uninsured problem, since more than 85 percent of the population remained content with their personal health coverage (Blendon 1997). Today, belief that the time for health reform has arrived is fueled moreover by the growth in support for change within the business community where concern over the cost of providing health insurance has deepened as economic conditions deteriorate. Employers confronted with declining profit margins and possible bankruptcy understandably are sympathetic to proposals freeing them from the cost of insuring their workers (Cohn 2007; Committee for Economic Development 2002).

Health providers previously opposed to health reform are undergoing a similar shift in thought because of the rising burden of uncompensated care from the growing number of unemployed workers. Physicians and hospitals together with other health care providers stand to benefit from universal coverage as more people would seek care and be able to pay their bills (Sack 2008; Dobias 2009).

Briefly put, the logic supporting national health insurance, or single-payer coverage as it is now euphemistically referred to, is as follows: inasmuch as health services tend to provide secure employment while at the same time constantly creating new jobs, higher spending, as discussed earlier, is desirable during a recession. Job creation helps revive depleted consumer spending and stimulate economic revival. National health insurance, for its part, could improve the economy by freeing up money that families can spend on other goods and services. The labor market also then benefits. When workers are freed from fear of losing coverage if they change jobs, they are more likely to switch to a more productive position and boost economic growth (Gruber 2009). Similar arguments pertain to universal coverage.

Health spending is justified additionally as a means for generating long-term benefits from investments in human capital and more efficient health services delivery. Thus health spending should be considered an asset to, rather than a drain on, the economy both in the short- and long-term benefits unleashed. Savings from investments in productivity and quality improvement moreover may be large enough to pay for much, if not all, of the cost of universal coverage (Cutler, Delong, and Marciarille 2008). While the current broad consensus for reform stirs confidence that long-sought changes are imminent, there are a number of troublesome issues lying beneath the surface that are not easily resolved.

Whether increasing the amount of money going to health care will in fact benefit the economy is questionable. By insisting on pushing ahead under bleak economic conditions, reform proponents risk abandoning prudence to emotion and may promise more than can be delivered. If, as is popularly assumed, social and political conditions actually do favor a major breakthrough in establishing universal coverage, any associated claims that the efficiency savings built into the program's design, notably investments in information technology and preventive medicine, will be enough to pay for the cost of increased coverage appears on close examination to be exaggerated (Pear 2008). Estimates made in the legislative phase about the future cost of social programs seldom are borne out in practice. Experience indicates that spending is far more likely to increase than decline.

A reduction or elimination of the uninsured problem is bound to increase demand for and consumption of health care services. Health care providers will be quick to meet this increased demand with an increased supply of products and services. Health care spending therefore will increase, making it all the harder to control as interest groups coalesce to block reductions and lobby for yet higher spending. It is politically unrealistic to expect otherwise. As astutely observed by Fuch, what is questionable spending to someone is someone else's income and that someone else will stoutly resist any attempt to take it away (Fuchs 2008: 1750).

Compromise Inescapable

It is unheard of for any major piece of legislation to emerge in its original form following congressional deliberations, especially when, as in the case of health reform, it is enshrouded in great controversy. No matter how well thought out and designed, the final shape of any health care proposal inevitably bears the influence of many competing interests without whose consent passage fails. Compromise is the essence of political decision-making.

Partisan and ideological differences must be accommodated in a system of government characterized by checks and balances and a division of powers. Thus any major expansion of health care coverage—a Democratic priority—will flounder unless provisions for tackling fast-growing health care costs—a top Republican concern—are included. Passage necessitates a balance between the social equity goals dear to liberal-minded reformers and the productivity and efficiency issues that concern their fiscally conservative colleagues.

Compromise is even more necessary in times when legislative power is not under the absolute control of a single party, or when a minority retains sufficient votes to block legislation through the power of filibuster. The same is true when ideological differences do not fall neatly along political party lines. Political parties typically consist of a mix of liberal, conservative, and moderate members whose divergent political and philosophical principles necessitate accommodation when the voting is close. Resolution of left and right wing differences is compounded as far as sectional and ideological factions exist within these categories, whose members often harbor deep-felt views not easily relinquished by entreaties to acquiesce for the benefit of party unity.

Additional negotiation and compromise stems from the complexity of the process whereby legislation moves through the Congress to the final enactment stage. The committees involved have an important voice in shaping outcomes. All health reform proposals are scrutinized by five different congressional committees, three of which are in the House and two in the Senate. (For a concise summary of the legislative process, see Shi and Singh 2008.)

It is rare that both the House and Senate versions of a legislative bill agree. Differences arising from these two legislative bodies must be submitted to a joint committee for negotiation and compromise. In light of the divisiveness marring congressional proceedings in recent decades, the chances of formulating the bipartisan sponsorship, which many analysts consider vital to the passage of meaningful health reform, are far from assured. (For a succinct description of the congressional complexities affecting health reform, see Iglehart 2009 and Fuchs 2009.)

Lobbyists also play an important role in affecting the outcome of legislation. Major spending bills invariably precipitate an outpouring of lobbyist activity that further tests the skill of political leadership to successfully steer a proposal through the legislative labyrinth. The prospect of a vast increase in the already large amount of money spent on health care is certain to attract the attention of vested interests. Profits from government-mandated spending are far more tempting than those derived from the uncertainties of market competition.

Like other groups dealing with Congress, health care providers and suppliers see campaign contributions and other financial favors as a way to gain access to policy makers. Naturally they want legislators to listen and act favorably on their agenda. The high cost of running for and remaining in office makes politicians willing participants. Practicality drives lobbyists' behavior. The recipients of lobbyist largesse generally transcend political and ideological affiliation. What matters most to lobbyists is the influence that individuals or organizations wield.

Lobbying activity also varies according to the timing of issues and their perceived importance to special interest sponsors. Since 2006, for example, the health industry has spent more on lobbying than any other sector of the economy, principally to defuse measures for cutting Medicare payments to hospitals, physicians, and other health providers (Center for Responsive Politics 2008).

An upsurge in lobbying is sure to parallel the legislative path of health reform. In 2008 there were 1,786 clients lobbying on health issues (Center for Responsive Politics 2008). It is unclear if this number will grow, but clearly the vested interests will become more deeply involved. The magnitude of the changes contemplated and their financial ramifications dwarf any health issue before the Congress since universal coverage was last attempted in the mid-1990s. It is not surprising therefore that the health care industry was the biggest lobbying force in Washington during the first half of 2009, a critical period during which various reform proposal were being formulated in key congressional committees, and that labor unions and other parties having a stake in the outcome also lobbied heavily (see Adamy and Williamson 2009: A1, A9). Accordingly the challenge of keeping core reform principles and objectives intact while managing a proposal through the legislative process is sure to be far more arduous than normal.

While there is no telling what to expect, one thing is certain—the plan that emerges will be the product of numerous negotiations and compromises. More specifically, interest groups in a position to block passage of universal coverage will not be predisposed to grant their approval should it entail any loss of income. Thus greater, rather than less, spending is the predictable price of enacting universal coverage. From this standpoint, attempting to address universal coverage and cost control as part of the same legislative package may be misadvised and unrealistic. It may prove wiser and more practical to confront them as two separate issues.

Assuming that the formidable legislative obstacles to health reform are successfully overcome, it may turn out in retrospect to have been the easy part. Because of complexities innate to health care, changing consumer and provider behavior to comply with legislative aims will require considerable effort. Altering long-ingrained behavioral patterns is the hard part.

Health Culture Encumbrances

Health care differs remarkably from other segments of the economy. It has the means to create its own demand, providing a rare instance where Say's Law actually applies. (Jean-Baptiste Say was a classical economist who held that recessions had become redundant because supply creates its own demand, a theory that prevailed until disproved by the Great Depression and the rise of Keynesian economics; see Galbraith and Salinger 1978: 18–19.) Most important, physicians are able to create demand for their services because of the authority they have over diagnosis and treatment. By virtue of this authority, they are in an unusually strong position to make or break reform objectives. Progress in improving efficiency and quality of care rests primarily therefore on physicians' support and cooperation.

Some of the more important standards governing physician behavior extend back to ancient Hellenic and Christian teachings. As initially embedded in these ancient teachings and continuing to the present day, a set of idealized norms has emerged on how physicians ought to conduct themselves when interacting with patients, and these norms are firmly immersed in the public mind. The same applies to hospitals. Whether or not they do so in practice, both medical and hospital professional associations profess to subscribe to idealized standards of conduct. Briefly stated, social expectations regarding physicians' behavior include an ethical obligation to preserve life, to place the welfare of patients ahead of self-gain, and to hold in confidence personal information acquired in the course of treatment (Edelstein 1943).

Knowledge obtained by long and demanding study, setting them apart from patients possessing little if any medical knowledge, inculcates in physicians a special authority, the exercise of which depends on trust in their competence and benevolence. Trust was and remains even more essential because of the emotional anxiety and fear patients experience in interpreting the significance of illness and the outcome of treatment. Illness confers on individuals a special state of vulnerability to physical and financial exploitation that, in the absence of trust, is a deterrent to the initiation of health care and effective treatment (Freidson 1970).

In order for a physician to instill trust, the patient must believe that the physician will do no harm. To this end, hospitals in the past often inscribed and displayed such assurance on a prominent wall or entryway to their facility. Although less true today as the result of advances in education and the flow of information, it was common in the past for the public to view physicians as a semi-priestly class dedicated to their patients' welfare and immune from temptations of money and self-aggrandizement.

Ethical principles extracted from the Hippocratic medicine were embodied in early Christian teachings and extended beyond curative medicine to include a special responsibility for the care of the incurably ill and dying, which laid the foundations for the growth of long-term care services and the hospice movement. Earlier on, the Greeks and other past civilizations believed health and fitness were paramount. The incurably ill and dying were viewed with opprobrium, as some sort of punishment for divine transgression or bad behavior. Later, the early Church elevated the sick and dying to a quasi-reverential status compelling devout followers to extend compassionate care and comfort. Religious instruction held all life to be sacred, as a gift from the Creator, and that it was unacceptable to end life by other than natural means once further ministration became hopeless. Meanwhile it was a moral imperative on the part of religious followers to do everything reasonable to preserve life. To this day abortion remains anathema within devout Christian circles.

Part of the justification for granting the sick a privileged status and entitlement to dignified and compassionate treatment derived from the conviction that they were victims of circumstances beyond their control and not responsible for what happened to them. From the Middle Ages onward, providing health care to the sick and terminally ill, independent of ability to pay and differences in social standing and lifestyle behavior, has been widely heralded as a hallmark of civilized society (Roemer 1960). The moral strength of this belief fuels contemporary political demands not only for national health insurance but for the inclusion of a constantly expanding range of covered health services. The doctrine that individuals have a universal right to adequate health care coverage also has its origin in religious social thought (Paterson 2004).

Although not recognized as such in today's more secular age, some of the more tenacious and polemical contemporary health policy and medical subjects have long historical connections, the most inflammatory of which bear a religious inheritance. Although typically presented in the context of humanitarian and egalitarian precepts, these controversies go beyond abortion to include physician-assisted suicide and denunciations of human rights abuses and capital punishment. Privacy of medical records also has long historical roots. Questions about whether too much or too little is being expended on the elderly, especially on end-of-life care, and whether long-term care services fail to receive their rightful share of resources relative to amounts spent on curative medicine are other issues traceable to early religious teachings.

Religious influence is also evident in the turmoil concerning whether not-for-profit hospitals should be eligible for tax benefits not permitted to for-profit rivals on the ground that not-for-profits no longer are performing charitable functions as originally intended (PriceWaterhouseCoopers 2006; Martinez and Carreyrou 2009). Belief in a charitable obligation to care for the poor was a major motivation in the initiation of the not-for-profit hospital movement that dominates the US hospital scene to this day.

During the Middle Ages what hospital care existed in much of Europe was largely run by religious orders. While most hospitals were secularized during the Reformation in England and elsewhere, they nevertheless bestowed a legacy of altruism and benevolence to their modern secular counterparts that underlies their tax status as charitable institutions. The not-for-profit hospital tradition is also a reflection of the early Church's admonitions against the profit motive and commercialization (Churchill 1958: 255–67).

Few contemporary public policy issues stir as much discord and acrimony as the role of profit in health care. Allegations that an inordinate share of private health insurance companies' profits are returned to investors and spent on excessive executive compensation are rife in the popular media. Controversy also surrounds charges that the federal government overpays private managed care firms participating in Medicare and that those firms care more about profits than meeting the health care needs of elderly clients (Cohn 2007).

As described previously, health insurance provided by private companies, whether nonprofit or for-profit, is 10 to 20 percent more costly than a public plan. Private insurers incur advertising and marketing expenses, are unable to benefit from economies of scale, and need to compensate investors, whereas a government plan has none of these disadvantages. Proponents of government-led universal coverage usually focus on these differences when dismissing market-based solutions as economically wasteful. Instead of benefiting private investors, they believe money going to profits would be better spent on making insurance more affordable for the poor and uninsured (Sherlock Company 2008; Physicians for a National Health Program 2007).

More broadly viewed, the commercialization of health care is rebuked for containing perverse incentives for the overproduction of health services, for exposing individuals to medically questionable and unnecessary care, and for denying the poor access to affordable quality care. Also commercialization is viewed as a major contributor to upwardly spiraling health care costs. Accordingly it has no place in a concept of health care as inherently a social good, and once again having strong religious and humanitarian connotations (e.g., see Physicians for a National Health Program 2006; Rice 1998; Himmelstein and Woolhandler 2008; Navarro 2008).

That ancient Hellenic and theological values dealing with access to health care and the insulation of the sick from exploitation have endured in one form or another down through the ages speaks to the significance of medicine for individual and social well-being. These values help illuminate how and why the profession of medicine acquired its special status. Because of the potential for patient abuse and harm when subjected to medical treatment, such as financial and sexual exploitation or poisoning, it was in society's interest to limit practice privileges. In return for abiding by a higher standard of conduct than found in commercial relationships, physicians were granted protection against market competition in the form of socially imposed restrictions on entry to medical practice and the privilege of self-regulation. Within the framework of this practical arrangement, the direct regulation of medicine was considered inadvisable. (On the social origins of professional sovereignty, see Starr 1982.)

Society also had a stake in controlling access to sick role privileges that exempt individuals from having to carry out their normal social responsibilities. In additional to the disruptive family and social effects from individuals wanting to escape unpleasant responsibilities by taking refuge in the sick role, there are also economic consequences in the form of job absenteeism and entitlement to government-funded cash benefits, such as worker's compensation and fraudulent medical expenses. (For a scholarly treatise on the social control function of medicine, see Parsons 1979.) In other words, laissez-faire medicine was assumed to be a danger to public health, and socially and economically dysfunctional.

Considerations such as these were instrumental in the decision made in the United States at the turn of the twentieth century—a time of competing medical schools and widespread quackery—to restrict the right to diagnose and treat to graduates of university-based allopathic schools of medicine. Competing schools of medicine, such as osteopathy, chiropractic naturopathy, and homeopathy, were marginalized as lacking a scientific basis (Shyrock 1967; Hudson 1978; Starr 1982). Whether these historic exclusionary practices remain justifiable today is worth reconsidering in light of the public's mounting reaction against orthodox medicine for being too expensive, and too depersonalized, and for treating patients as an assemblage of body parts rather than holistically. The options available for alleviating physician shortages in such areas as obstetrics and primary care remain limited, even though there has been a recent relaxation of licensing and regulatory restrictions over authority to diagnose and treat, and even though qualified substitutes exist such as nurse practitioners, nurse midwives, and nurse anesthetists (e.g., see Reeves et al. 2004; Moore 2000).

Because of differences in length and cost of education, effective use of substitute medical personnel would help lower the cost of routine health care while improving access to basic services among impoverished and medically underserved areas. Lifting restrictions on the use of nurse practitioners, for instance, would free physicians now engaged in primary care to concentrate on intellectually and professionally more challenging medical responsibilities while simultaneously improving their incomes. Not only is this a better use of expensive personnel, but it acknowledges a major cause of why it is so difficult to attract medical school graduates into primary care.

Invidious status distinctions rooted in old exclusionary policies moreover limit the application of inexpensive alternatives in favor of costly high-technology medical interventions. Treatments emphasizing dietary and lifestyle changes, for example, are said to have the potential to prevent up to 90 percent of all heart disease and thus sharply reduce the need for costly coronary angioplasty and bypass procedures, amounting to around $100 billion in annual spending (Chopra, Ornish, and Weil 2009; Majid 2004).

Strictly speaking, self-regulation is something less than an unrestricted right. The legal aspects of medical practice, including the disciplining of malpractice and other errant behavior, are a state government responsibility (Derbyshire 1969). However, state regulation generally has been overly responsive to the interest of the medical profession Apart from bureaucrats succumbing to the homage factor commanded by medicine during its more elevated status in earlier years, medical lobbyists so successfully co-opt key legislative and executive agencies that, practically speaking, they serve as proxies for the medical profession (Public Citizen 2006). A manifestation of this is that health care is organized more for the convenience of physicians and other health providers than for the convenience of patients. As noted by Herzlinger, instead of integrated health care teams and services located on a single site, treatment is provided by many different specialists requiring separate appointments and travel to different offices and sites (Herzlinger 2007).

Strong influence of regulatory bodies by parties under their scrutiny is not uncommon. It is a serious problem affecting all regulatory agencies (Stigler 1971). Underfunding and understaffing of state regulatory bodies is yet another issue. However, the value of spending to reinvigorate and improve state regulatory agencies appears problematic. The persistence of problems such as the maldistribution of physicians among states and the administrative-legal barriers curtailing use of telemedicine for bringing quality health care into medically underserved areas suggests that state regulation itself is part of the problem. State regulation is an anachronism when viewed in terms of the barriers to physician interstate mobility and telemedicine applications. Furthermore lack of uniform national standards and regulations sows confusion and subjects citizens to different standards of medical accountability depending on where they live.

Looked at from a historical perspective, freedom from outside interference in the practice of medicine was not a privilege granted idly. Rather, it more appropriately represented a practical concession to the unpredictability of disease and medical treatment. The natural history of disease is such that susceptibility to and severity of illness varies among individuals, as does their responsiveness to treatment. Thus patterns normally found in the health statistics of large populations do not apply at the patient level. For this reason only physicians familiar with a patient's medical and personal history were believed to be qualified to determine what constitutes optimal treatment.

In effect physicians were free to exercise their professional judgment without having to worry about being second-guessed by persons unqualified in medicine. This accounts for the medical profession's historic opposition to third-party intrusion and, in particular, why management has long been considered the enemy of good patient care. Medical revulsion against the growth of corporate hospital chains and managed care firms is based on this very point. (For a seminal article on this theme, see Relman 1980.)

Preservation of clinical autonomy indeed dominated the politics of organized medicine throughout the past century and continues to do so today. At the time of Medicare's enactment in the mid-1960s the American Medical Association so vehemently opposed what it feared might challenge the survival of solo, fee-for-service medicine that the federal government formally pledged not to interfere with the practice of medicine in order to get the legislation through Congress (Harris 1966). This concession has had long-term consequences as evidenced in today's concern over the sustainability of Medicare financing. Clinical autonomy is at the heart of the financial and quality control problems now besetting Medicare, and a primary reason why it has been so hard to bring its spending under control. Indeed the primacy given to clinical autonomy within the medical profession points to why physicians continue to practice in small-sized groups. It also explains their hostility toward the concept of managed care and efforts to subject clinical decision-making to oversight and evaluation by anyone other than physicians.

In general, the public shares these same professional values and endorses fee-for-service and freedom-of-choice programs. They repudiate managed care and efficiency reforms that attempt to place limits on the availability of services failing to meet cost-effectiveness criteria. Successful health reform hinges on whether public opinion can be swayed to accept changes in physician reimbursement and patient's freedom of choice, but this will not be easily accomplished. Individuals are highly reluctant to give up what they consider to be of benefit to themselves. Whereas all occupations and social institutions have experienced a steep decline in public confidence and esteem in recent decades, the medical profession continues to be held in relatively high regard despite the fall it too has suffered in the public trust it once enjoyed. Physicians now rank in fifth place, behind teachers and druggists (Romano 2005). Nevertheless, shared medical and public values comprise a formidable political alliance that remains slow to accept the need for broad-scale health care reform. Regardless of how the medical profession is viewed, most individuals retain considerable confidence in their personal physician and satisfaction with their care (Mechanic 2006).

Market Inapplicability

Along with the continuing influence of historic cultural values, health care differs from other industries in the extent to which the conventional rules of market competition are believed to be inapplicable. While

not all economists agree with this assertion, it nevertheless has dominated health reform deliberations in the post–World War II era and is
considered by many to be an unalterable distinction. In brief, serious
imperfections in the structure of the health market are said to prevent
market competition from promoting efficiency and an optimal allocation resources (Arrow 1963; Klarman 1965; Fuchs 1972: 3–12).

First, health care does not fit the definition of a normal commodity.
Rather, it is an intangible product characterized by considerable uncertainty over what is received when purchasing a service. At best, one is
buying an unknown, but hopefully substantial, reduction in the probability of serious illness, disability, and premature death. Where matters
of illness and medical treatment are involved, there are no guarantees.

A second distinction is that consumer decision-making is impaired
by anxiety and fear over the possibility of serious disability and premature death to the point that emotion rather than rationality directs an
individual's actions. This problem is complicated by the individual's
disadvantage in having to rely on medical experts because of an inadequate personal understanding of medical knowledge. Decision-making
authority consequently falls heavily on physicians. Due to the asym-
metry of information, individuals seeking health care undergo a form
of decision-making paralysis that puts them in a subordinate and dependent position. Having initiated health care, an individual can only
hope that the physician consulted is technically competent and ethically
disposed to act with the patient's welfare in mind.

In recognition of the constraints on consumer sovereignty, the courts
ruled in the mid-1970s that the relationship between patients and physicians does not fit the rules applied to commercial transactions (Annas 1998). Rather than an arm's-length business arrangement, it is a
trust-based relationship in which the physician assumes fiduciary responsibilities. Thus the practice of medicine is neither a business nor
a trade, but one in which the physician serves as an advocate for the
patient.

Another difference centers on the social restrictions placed on the
authority to diagnose and treat illness. Licensure requirements in the
United States limit the practice of medicine to individuals completing
lengthy medical education and postgraduate training requirements.
Although somewhat liberalized in recent decades, legal authority to
prescribe medicines and to conduct surgery is still closely confined to
graduates of allopathic medical schools. With the major exception of os-
teopathic physicians who were granted co-equal status in the 1960s and
who comprise a small minority of physicians, practitioners graduating

from non-allopathic programs, such as those related to the practice of chiropractic and homeopathic medicine, have far more limited powers. As the result of restrictions over entry into medical practice, physicians enjoy unusual freedom to determine the prices they charge under fee-for-service reimbursement while possessing an ability to create their own demand.

Finally, the role played by third-party payers (private insurers and government) alters the normal buyer–seller relationship. Because most consumers of health care are largely insulated from directly paying for the services they use, health care is generally perceived as an unlimited free good having all the associated connotations for wasteful spending. This assumption is the outgrowth of policies designed initially to maintain household financial security by insuring consumers against the high cost of serious illness. It was later liberalized to encourage the early initiation for routine medical services

Early public policy in support of health insurance was based on the rationale that in contrast to other goods and services, it was hard for individuals to budget for health care due to the unpredictability of illness, both in terms of its occurrence and severity, following which it was impossible to predict the cost and outcome of treatment. Consequently protecting individuals from the cost of health care insurance has disconnected them from the ordinary consumer's sensitivity to the price of purchasing decisions and set in motion a hard to contain inflationary dynamic (PriceWaterhouseCoopers 2005).

Social Good Status

As construed by proponents of government financing, health care fails the test of a commercial commodity for reasons that go beyond the above-mentioned market imperfections. To them, it better fits the description of a social good (e.g., see Krugman and Walls 2006). First and foremost, access to health care is an indispensable element for the construction of social harmony. Apart from the moral obligation civilized societies have to care for the poor, the sick, the infirm, and the dying, there are a number of practical reasons for doing so. While normally subordinated to the moral rationale and mentioned less frequently, there are other social benefits.

By assuring individuals that they are valued by their community, access to high-quality health care contributes to their self-esteem and emotional and mental health. A healthy and happy population in turn helps build social solidarity through the amelioration of envy and despondency over disparities in health care. When well maintained, the resulting social and political stability creates an environment favorable to long-term investment and economic growth (e.g., see Wilkinsong 1997).

Other community benefits accrue from investments in communicable disease control and public health measures, together with spending on maternal and child health. Spending on infant and children's health, in particular, has positive long-term labor force benefits. Healthier children are better able to access educational opportunities that lead to more skilled and productive workers. Properly financed and organized health care moreover supports economic productivity and growth by lowering sickness-related job absenteeism while at the same time reducing social expenditures for sick-leave pay, worker's compensation, and social security disability payments (e.g., see Davis 2005). National security and military preparedness is a not a commonly recognized but important benefit. Of the young men drafted into the military in 1962, 50 percent were rejected for medical conditions that were considered treatable and correctable, a finding that influenced the improved coverage of children in the Medicaid program (Rosenbaum 2005).

Finally, health-related employment is yet another benefit of health spending. Regardless of economic conditions, the health sector is an important source of high-status jobs for the upwardly mobile offspring of low- and middle-income families and, provides stable employment for semi-skilled and low-skilled workers. Hospitals and long-term care facilities often serve as one of the few remaining employers of unskilled workers in economically decimated inner cities and rural areas.

Redemptive Power of National Health Insurance

Government-financed health care may not be the ultimate panacea for the problems now besetting health care but advocates nevertheless consider it far superior to the alternatives. Universal coverage and the removal of price and income barriers to the early initiation of physician and hospital services not only fulfill health care's core humanitarian-egalitarian purpose but provide a way for the nation to save money. Within the contemporary political context of health reform, the potential for saving money has been elevated to become a persuasive utilitarian argument for enactment of national health insurance or a single-payer system.

Although not always overt, this assertion rests on several major propositions. First, spending assuredly will increase following passage of universal free care but will level off as the backlog of unmet medical needs are satisfied. Spending should decline once the benefits of investments in disease prevention and health maintenance start to appear. Second, discounts obtained by government as a large buyer of pharmaceuticals, and other health supplies and equipment will generate substantial savings. Third, additional savings will result from reductions in medical costs as a consequence of government-mandated controls. Such controls include limiting the amount health providers charge for services, placing a ceiling on executive compensation, subjecting hospitals and physicians to fixed operating budgets, and discontinuing payments for treatments failing cost-effectiveness evaluation. England is often cited in this regard as an outstanding example of how subjecting health providers to fixed budgets and limiting the diffusion of medical innovations to those meeting rigorous evaluative criteria succeed in containing health spending growth. As a percentage of GDP, England spends less on health care than any other highly developed country (e.g., see Davis 2008).

In keeping with these beliefs, the Obama administration contends that passage of its universal coverage plan will produce substantial savings rather than add to the government's serious financial problems. Returns from disease prevention programs and improvements in the treatment of costly chronic conditions, like hypertension, heart disease, diabetes, and asthma, supposedly will produce savings of $80 billion per year. Another $80 billion is anticipated in efficiency savings from investments in information technology and mass purchasing (Enthoven 2008). If politically useful for assuaging concerns over affordability of universal coverage in light of the severity of the nation's financial problems, these numbers nevertheless stretch the credulity of seasoned health care observers, particularly since there is no mention of using centralized controls or changes in the way health care is organized and delivered (Enthoven 2008).

Finally, there is a fourth proposition that is perhaps the most compelling to universal coverage proponents—the elimination of social and economic health disparities. As discussed later, it is equally doubtful, given the experience of other countries, whether health status difference among geographic, socioeconomic, racial, and ethnic groups can be eradicated solely through the infusion of money for health services given the interplay of other, if not more important, factors (Wilkinson 1997).

Summary

The obstacles standing in the way of change described previously suggest that comprehensive health reform will follow a labored path. While the economic calamity now gripping the nation may indeed open the way to politically stalled health policy objectives, the opportunities created, in all likelihood, will be much smaller than envisioned. Health care comprises almost 17 percent of a giant-sized national economy. It is characterized by unmatched complexity and composed of powerful interest groups with a long history of bending change to their advantage. With this in mind, the enormity of the task becomes staggering.

The risk in wholesale health reform is that a bad situation inadvertently is made worse. The revisions and compromises that inevitably arise in the legislative process when combined with health care's complexity may result in something less than intended. The chances of bipartisan cooperation require an inferential leap given the bitter partisan and ideological strife characteristic of Washington politics in recent years. Even if the original objectives emerge intact, there is the omnipresent danger of unintended consequences to consider. (For an instructive discussion of the political difficulties involved in forming successful coalitions for comprehensive reform, see Aaron 1996.)

The passage of universal coverage legislation will in itself be a formidable test of the fortitude and resourcefulness of those entrusted with the project. Rather than add to the already high controversy encumbering the attainment of universal coverage, political prudence points to a more cautious approach that deals with other equally controversial objectives, such as cost containment and quality improvement, separately and incrementally. If infrastructure failings are not corrected first, then investing additional large sums in health care will be ineffective and therefore wasteful. Progress on any health reform objective is bound to be tedious inasmuch as behavioral standards and expectations shaping physician behavior are deeply immersed in a culture of professional sovereignty and clinical autonomy that is highly resistant to change. Failure to appreciate the difficulty in modifying physician and patient behavior explains in large part why earlier attempts at cost containment and managed care failed.

3   Contemporary Challenges

Overcoming resistance to health reform that is embedded in the culture of health care presents a major challenge to the possibility of bringing health spending under control in a manner that reconciles competing demands for economy and social justice. This tension is foremost in decisions that will have to be made regarding the disproportionate share of health expenditures directed to individuals at the extremes of the life cycle. It is inevitable therefore that economy-minded policy makers will focus their attention on the value of resources committed to individuals at the end of life and to newborns requiring expensive intensive neonatal and life-long health and social support services. These two groups account for close to 40 percent of all health spending, and nearly one-third of all Medicare spending occurs in the last six months of life. (Cutler and Meara 2009; Lubitz and Riley 1993).

The technology of medicine today is very sophisticated but also very expensive. What Medicare now spends on drugs is illustrative. Mainly due to the cost of new drugs for the treatment of cancer, Medicare spending on medical prescriptions rose from $3 billion in 1997 to $11 billion in 2004—an increase of 267 percent. In comparison, overall Medicare spending rose by only 47 percent (Bach 2009). New drug therapies contain the power to turn fatal conditions into chronic disorders but at costs that can approach $50,000 to $100,000 a year (Lee and Emanuel 2008).

Conditions have reached the stage where the nation, despite its wealth, cannot continue to fund the best that medicine can provide to all members of the population. Financial exigencies inexorably will steer policy makers to differentiate spending in terms of investment and consumption criteria. Flexibility for doing so, however, will be constrained by ethical and moral values that are deeply embedded in health culture. Attitudes toward abortion and end-of-life care therefore have an important bearing on the scope for cost containment. There is no doubt that the terminal elderly and infants requiring intensive neonatal care benefit considerably from medical treatment in terms of enhanced quality of life. But the return to society is ambiguous from the standpoint of the effects on economic productivity and wealth creation, since the individuals in these categories have little or no connection to the labor force.

Beyond these issues this chapter presents other cultural factors that are sure to influence the outcome of health reforms. In this regard historic health-culture suspicions against the application of market forces are a major deterrent to the formation of creative public-private partnerships that can enable the federal government to solve the uninsured problem and other health reform goals without exacerbating already severely overextended financial capabilities.

In addition to helping the government better manage its finances, market forces are revealed that are useful for circumventing interest groups opposed to health reform and for curbing the inflationary dynamic inherent in third-party fee-for-service reimbursement. The extent to which consumers can be enlisted in cost containment and quality improvement initiatives depends on altering the perception of health care as a free good along with the changing the belief that individuals are incapable of making intelligent medical decisions free of medical paternalism.

Finally, conventional wisdom denial of the possibility that health care fits the definition of a consumer good is rejected as a shibboleth that masks recognition of a vibrant private-pay health care market for elective services along with features of primary care services that are amenable to private payment.

Evolution of Quality of Life Values

It is a testimony to the staying power of health care values entwined in early Hellenic and Christian teachings that they have endured throughout the ages, but their influence clearly is waning as traditional social mores are giving way to changes in social expectations and conditions of modern living. Advances in mass education, higher living standards, and population aging, together with a secular outlook on the value of life, are radically modifying attitudes toward existence and survival.

Although life itself is no less valued, today's emphasis is on the quality of life rather than its preservation. Incurable suffering, survival under conditions of diminished mental and physical capacity for independent living, and loss of personal dignity are no longer embraced as a state of divine grace as they were by previous generations. Increasingly the quality of life is valued more than longevity itself. A condition of equilibrium between the two remains the aspired ideal. But failing that, the qualitative aspects take precedence. This is especially true of the elderly whose numbers are increasing as the result of improvements in medicine and living standards. For a growing number of today's elderly, death is not feared so much as incurable pain, disability, and the loss of capacity for independent living. As the perceived quality of life declines, suicide becomes a more acceptable alternative.

To be sure, improvements in palliative medicine have done much to ameliorate unbearable anxiety over physical and emotional suffering, thereby lessening the appeal of suicide as a means of escape. Nevertheless, the possibility of diminished mental capacity or languishing in an unpredictably long vegetative state causes anxiety. This explains why advance legal directives have become a common practice in planning for individual health and medical contingencies as a way of avoiding unacceptable end-of-life conditions.

For many, alleviating family emotional and financial strains, and lessening the burden on society from the cost of institutional care once individual and family resources are exhausted, are the socially responsible things to do. In the absence of a clear directive, withdrawal of life support care for ostensibly permanently brain-dead individuals is, to the consternation of loved ones seeking a merciful end on their behalf, mired in legal complexity and controversy. While not impossible, permission to withdraw life support in such cases involves lengthy and costly legal delays. Few incidents illustrate this as dramatically as the Terry Schiavo case that dominated the national media a few years ago (Didion 2005; Hampton and Emanuel 2005).

Abortion

Although fraught with controversy, attitudes toward abortion are similarly changing as parents increasingly weigh the consequences of bringing children into the world that, because of the severity of mental and/ or physical disability, are medically determined incapable of becoming independent adults or are destined for an unacceptably low quality of life. The burden of providing custodial care in the family household weighs heavily on parental decisions. The prospect of an offspring having to adjust to an institutional facility once family members are no longer able to care for them at home, whether due to physical and emotional exhaustion or advancing age and mortality, compounds the dilemma. (For a good description of the stressful choices parents encounter when prenatal testing identifies genetic maladies and rare medical conditions, see Naik 2008: A1, A18.)

As attested by the objections of right-to-life supporters, not everyone agrees that abortion ought to be a choice in such instances, but given that the dissenters bear few if any of the personal costs of such a decision, public opinion generally sides with parental choice. In addition to sympathy for the plight of affected parents and larger humanitarian considerations, public opinion also reflects in part mounting unease over the long-term social services costs involved in caring for individuals incapable of self-support, particularly in instances where institutionalization is a high probability.

More controversial yet, is the issue of whether abortion should be used as a social policy instrument for combating unwanted pregnancies. Nearly half of all pregnancies in the United States are unintended. Of these, 40 percent are aborted. Among all pregnancies—miscarriages excluded—roughly one-fifth end in abortion. Each year about 2 percent of women aged 15 to 44 have an abortion, and close to half of them have had at least one previously (Guttmacher Institute 2008).

While, due to the improved use of contraceptives, the abortion rate has declined somewhat in recent years to 25 percent below its all-time high of 1.6 million in 1990, there were still 1.2 million abortions performed in 2005 (Guttmacher Institute Media Center 2008). Whether, and to what extent, more informed use of contraceptives can lower abortion numbers below the current rate is questionable. Over half of women receiving an abortion report having used a contraceptive method (mainly condoms or pills) during the month they became pregnant. However, newer methods requiring less frequent application and those that provide longer term protection may prove more successful.

Unwed teenage pregnancy and abortion is an especially volatile mix, for it encapsulates a number of other controversial and politically sensitive issues involving race and strategies for attacking poverty. While many, if not most, teenage mothers genuinely want children, they typically are not equipped in terms of maturity, education, and material well-being to properly care for them. So both they and their children become trapped in a downward cycle of deprivation and poverty—ending too often in multigenerational dependency on government welfare programs. (For an analysis of the relationship of illegitimacy, poverty, and welfare, see Bane 1994 and Moynihan 1965.)

In short, socioeconomic circumstances typically are nonconducive to good childhood development. The fact that out-of-wedlock teenage births are disproportionately associated with low-income minority women adds to this bleak prognosis, as does discrimination to the difficulty of becoming financially self-sufficient. Exceptions notwithstanding, this scenario is considered the common pattern.

The cost to society, in terms of individuals' inability to maintain steady employment beyond minimum wage levels, chronic unemployment, antisocial behaviors, and the broad array of social welfare support services, is a common reason given for condoning teenage abortion. Analyses conducted in the late 1980s indicated that for every tax dollar spent to pay for abortions for poor women governments save around four dollars from resulting lower medical and welfare expenditures. The net savings for the nation as a whole over a two-year period if abortions were publicly funded in every state was estimated at close to $340 million (Torres et al. 1986).

Although marriage and the postponement of children until the completion of education may be a better way to reduce poverty in this group, changing behavior is far more difficult and it entails costly long-term strategies. If less effective in the end, abortion is accepted as an expedient short-term measure. There is a close correlation of abortion to marital status, education, and poverty. It is reflected in the facts that teenage women account for 17 percent of all abortion procedures, single women living below the federal poverty line are more than four times likely to have an abortion than their higher income counterparts, and women living below the poverty line are nearly four times as likely to have an unintended pregnancy than women who are not poor (Guttmacher Institute 2008).

Despite legalization and broad-based social acceptance, abortion remains a highly contentious issue among persons subscribing to right-to-life doctrines and the ascription of legal rights to the unborn. Few social policy disputes match the intensity of emotion stirred by the abortion issue. It is a major contributor to the decade's-long culture wars bedeviling the nation's political tranquility. Confrontations between pro- and anti-abortion groups have been known to turn violent. Abortion opponents are endlessly persevering. In addition to constant legal challenges, impassioned anti-abortion sentiment is expressed in numerous tactics designed to weaken the resolve of proponents by making life difficult for women seeking abortion and for medical staff conducting the procedure.

At just what point in the pregnancy cycle life is believed to begin is the heart of the dispute. Opinions range from the onset of conception to the beginning and the end of the third trimester. This lack of consensus adds to the controversy over abortion. It also underlies the disputes over the moral and legal status of stem cell research using fetal tissue. Despite vociferous and unyielding views to the contrary, abortion commands both a firm legal standing and the endorsement of the American Medical Association (AMA), largely on the grounds that a fetus is not a human being. However, abortion remains a matter of dissension within the provider community as a number of physicians and hospitals harbor religious objections that, until recently, have been respected by the federal government but now are being reconsidered amid intensive moral controversy. (For a concise review of the issues, see Cantor 2009.)

Physician-Assisted Suicide

Physician-assisted suicide for the terminally ill is a more ambiguous issue in that it is not nationally legalized and does not have the support of the medical establishment. Unlike abortion where the definition of life is disputable, it clearly involves the taking of a human life. Therefore organized medicine is reluctant to sanction it. Taking life, while at the same time protecting life, undermines medical authority and the trust essential to the physician–patient relationship (AMA 2008).

In light of improvements in palliative care and pain management, the American Medical Association contends that providing responsible alternative treatment to ending life removes the need for euthanasia. While true that many physicians remain poorly trained in palliative medicine and pain management, competence is fast spreading. Where medical practice fails, hospice care, which has led the way in enlightened end-of-life medical and psychological services, is an excellent alternative in many communities.

Nevertheless, public support for physician assistance in terminating end-of-life suffering and indignities appears strong and growing. Although some thirty-five states have criminalized mercy killing, this has not dissuaded voters in Oregon from legalizing physician-assisted suicide and one can anticipate that interest in aid-in-dying will not abate. Although defeated in recent ballot measures undertaken in Washington, California, and Maine, the winning margins were small—proponents acquired from 46 to 49 percent of the vote. Michigan was an exception. Voters there defeated physician-assisted suicide by a margin of 29 percent. On the other hand, in the period 1994 through 2007 there were ninety failed legislative proposals in twenty-three states (International Task Force on Euthanasia and Assisted Suicide 2009). Like abortion, physician-assisted suicide is caught in the tensions between traditional and contemporary values.

Anti-market Bias

As previously said, anti-market bias is deeply entrenched in health care, the roots of which extend back over two millennia. Doctrines proclaiming free health care as a fundamental human right also stem from this legacy. Anti-market bias remains very much alive in the current debate over health reform, as evident in the convictions energizing proponents of taxpayer-financed comprehensive universal health coverage or a single-payer system

The emotional intensity with which government financing and control is seen as the ultimate solution to the uninsured problem and related issues of quality improvement and cost containment is a deterrent to dispassionate discussion and objective analysis. It blinds advocates to the possibility that market-based strategies can play a constructive role in health reform. The harm to sound decision-making that occurs when emotion prevails over reason is compounded when, as often occurs, ideologues holding different convictions clash. A stalemate is the consequence. Advocates for the penultimate powers of market competition are no less unreasonable.

Ideological intransigence and conflict rank among some of the more important reasons why past attempts at health reform have failed. They are factors in the current search for practical means for overcoming opposition to higher efficiency and quality control standards. Most important, strong anti-market sentiment hampers efforts to expand coverage of the uninsured in a way that minimizes the cost to government. This occurs at a time when public finances are under great duress because of the vast outlay of federal dollars required to mitigate the effects of the greatest economic collapse the nation has experienced since the Great Depression.

The massive borrowing necessary for dealing with the economic crisis has resulted in the biggest federal deficit in the past half century, estimated to total more than 12 percent of GDP in 2009—a deficit level unseen since World War II (see Gale and Auerbach 2009). The new spending required to revive the economy will vastly add to the federal debt in the next few years to the point where the nation's credit rating may be jeopardized. It is projected by Moody's Investors Service that the total public debt as a percentage of GDP will jump from around 40 percent in 2008 to over 60 percent by 2010. The Congressional Budget Office believes it may reach 80 percent by 2019. Dealing with debt of such magnitude is difficult. Raising taxes to repay the debt or manipulating the economy using methods like inflation and devalued currency creates a host of other hard to resolve problems (Congressional Budget Office 2009; Rappaport 2009).

When translated to the personal level, the ramification is staggering. If combined with the size of unfunded future payments for Social Security, Medicare, and Medicaid, the current deficit means that every American bears a financial burden of $184,000—if federal spending is not contained and nothing is done to address the unfunded entitlement problem (Peter G. Peterson Foundation 2009).

Hidden Pragmatism of Market Competition

Intransigence on the part of health providers, insurers, and other health sector interests has, as mentioned earlier, been the downfall of previous attempts at large-scale health reform. These vested interests threatened by change are remarkably adroit at circumventing legislative actions and redirecting planning and regulatory controls to their advantage. To assume that this will change is folly. Political resolution of differences has fallen short in the past. Whether this time around the political climate is more auspicious is speculative. But should a political solution fail once again, market dynamics may prove to be more successful.

Improvements occur faster and with less acrimony when left to market competition than if the same objectives are sought through legislative edict or planning regulations when dealing with obstinate interest group opposition. Responsibility for resisted change is depersonalized and outcomes are determined by competition in which involved parties assume they have an opportunity to affect their own fate. In comparison, change occurs more slowly when pursued through the imposition of government directives. Political decision-making is inherently fraught with complexities and delays and subject to lengthy legal challenges instigated by disaffected or dispossessed interests (Battistella 1997).

In short, market competition works better because it depoliticizes responsibility for decision-making. Outcomes are determined by a proverbial invisible hand. Skeptics may deprecate this as an illusion, but here may be an instance where perception is reality. Market competition moreover is noted for its ability to stimulate efficiency and quality improvements. It does this by forcing providers to compete against one another and by capturing the power of self-interest in pursuit of market share and profits.

Within a competitive environment prosperity and survival rests on outperforming one's rivals when dealing with informed buyers who are motivated to obtain the best service at the lowest price. Those providers who fail to supply efficient services or superior products suffer financially and risk failure. Those who succeed prosper. Industrywide performance standards are upgraded in the process. Government, on the contrary, is purposely inefficient. It is designed to slow the pace of change that is disruptive to individual rights and social stability. It is not surprising therefore that some of the earliest breakthroughs in overcoming provider barriers to efficiency and quality improvements stemmed mainly from private-sector leadership. (For examples, see Sloan 2000.)

Although highly controversial and repudiated as a threat to core health values, publicly traded hospital firms pioneered health industry horizontal and vertical integration. They applied modern corporate and managerial methods that are now widely emulated among not-for-profit hospitals to the extent that the differences between profit and not-for-profit hospitals are miniscule. Publicly traded hospital chains also were first to treat hospital staff as a variable rather than fixed cost. (For a discussion of health sector opposition to corporatization, see Starr 1982.)

As the principal purchasers of health services, employers, though reluctant to do so historically, have been using their purchasing power more aggressively over the past several decades to influence providers to supply efficient and quality services and products. Large corporations seeking greater value for their employee health outlays are in the forefront of the movement to introduce modern managerial practices. They leverage their resources and size to overcome health providers' resistance to advanced efficiency and quality improvement methods such as management information technology, performance-based compensation, transparent price and quality reporting, electronic medical records, medical report cards, and evidence-based medical standards. Their efforts to spur reforms have been most effective when done in concert with other large firms and groups, and structured as consortia such as the Leapfrog Group and Bridges to Excellence. (For a description of these two groups, see The Leapfrog Group 2009.)

Free-Good Psychology

Corporate and government use of purchasing power has had minimal effect on slowing the pace of health spending; the managed care initiatives they supported in the mid-1990s were a notable but temporary exception. While they pay for most of the nation's health care, they do not control the day-to-day utilization decisions that cumulatively translate into health spending totals—others do.

These others are individuals who have little interest in the cost of services largely because they do not pay for the charges. Since 1960 the share of health costs paid for out of pocket has declined from nearly half to just under 13 percent (Kirkegaard 2009). Employers and government pay all or most of the bills. It is unrealistic to expect that individuals will exhibit the same attentiveness to cost when spending someone else's money as compared to their own.

Inflationary health spending is unlikely to subside unless and until individuals are empowered to act as prudent consumers. The conditions required for this to happen are, first, the consumer needs to be intimately involved in paying for the cost of their care rather than relegating payment to a third party and, second, consumers need access to user-friendly reliable price and quality information on specific providers to enable knowledgeable comparisons. Recent gains in provider transparency are helpful but more needs to be done in expanding the scope and usefulness of data for guiding consumer choice.

Individuals need to abandon the passive-submissive patient role and act more assertively to get the best-priced quality care. Among any other questions, they routinely should ask their health providers the following: How much will this cost? Is there a less expensive alternative? What is the likely benefit from a proposed treatment? Do I need all of the recommended treatment? And what are the associated risks? The positive effects of this empowerment would be even greater if individuals were made partners in cost containment by permitting them to share in any savings, thereby unleashing the full motivational power of self-interest. (Further discussion on individuals and their role in cost containment can be found in chapter 6.)

Medical Paternalism

The physician–patient relationship today bears a much diminished relationship compared to what it used to be. Physicians no longer command the same authoritarian and semi-priestly status of earlier years. Higher education and medical information levels diminish the need for patients to depend entirely on medical authority. Accordingly they have become less acquiescent and submissive. To be sure, physicians continue to be held in high regard, but without the mystique and awe commanded when medicine was more of a mystery to an uninformed public. Whereas patients formerly tended to rely totally on physicians to make medical decisions on their behalf and complied without question to medical authority, a more highly educated public and the greater availability of user-friendly medical information enables them to be more independent and assertive in matters concerning their health treatment choices.

Greater transparency of clinical data together with information on the quality and cost of hospital and physician services on a provider specific basis, all of which is easily accessible on the Internet and in consumer information publications, underlies the process whereby patients are being transformed into consumers (for more on this transformation, see Herzlinger 1997). Thus shopping around for the best medical care is becoming the norm, and the seeking of second opinions, something eschewed in the past by physicians as errant patient behavior, is now openly encouraged and a synonym for rational behavior.

As consumers, individuals now want to know more about the various treatment alternatives available to them along with the latest evidence on the benefits and risks involved. Such behavior differs markedly, of course, from the old physician–patient model in which medical information was considered beyond the comprehension of laypersons and anxiety over the seriousness of symptoms rendered individuals incapable of reliably acting on their own behalf.

That principles of consumer-directed care are redefining the physician–patient relationship coincides with a shift in disease patterns that has introduced greater uncertainty in clinical decision-making. Previously physicians treated predominately acute disorders where treatment was characterized by a high degree of medical consensus. Now chronic degenerative disorders dominate physicians' attention. These conditions are typically marked by the availability of multiple treatment choices and uncertainty over which one best fits a patient's particular situation and needs.

Acute conditions are marked by sudden dramatic onset, have a single cause, and lend themselves to treatment by a single physician. In comparison, chronic conditions develop slowly and insidiously, have complex and frequently multiple causes, and are best treated with multidisciplinary, multiprofessional health care teams. The many alternatives for dealing with back pain are indicative of the ambiguity and uncertainty in the treatment of chronic conditions, as are the multiple choices for the treatment of breast and prostate cancers. Eliciting patients as partners in decision-making is a sensible thing to do under conditions of clinical uncertainty. Individuals who participate in the choice of treatment method are apt to be more highly motivated in adhering to medical instructions and therapeutic protocol, thereby facilitating better outcomes.

Noncompliance is a big problem, particularly in connection with the treatment of chronic illness. Half of patients fail to follow physicians' instruction or take medicines as prescribed. Failure to do so results in nearly one-quarter of all nursing home admissions, one-tenth of hospital admissions, and countless extra office visits, tests, and procedures. Noncompliance among cardiac patients is said to cause 125,000 annual deaths (Vermeire et al. 2001; Landro 2005: D9; Orszag 2008). Noncompliance underscores the physician's dilemma, and it is a seldom-mentioned dimension of quality improvement. Quality of care and favorable outcomes is a shared physician–patient responsibility. Without the patient's cooperation, the best of treatment can go wrong. It is important therefore that initiatives for quality improvement also address patient behavior (Vermeire et al. 2001; Landro 2005: D9). Shared decision-making can also help save money. When the choices available to patients are made clear, they tend to prefer less invasive and less expensive treatments than they otherwise would.

Enlisting patients as partners in medical treatment is also a useful means for reducing the incidence of litigation and malpractice claims. Having participated in the treatment decision in which the benefits and risks of alternatives are reviewed and assessed, individuals are psychologically less inclined to seek legal recourse when treatment fails to work as anticipated. In the new consumer-driven era, physicians and hospitals will find it ever more difficult to shelter what they do from public scrutiny. Self-monitoring, self-regulation, and self-reporting clearly are on the wane. There is no evading public scrutiny in the modern information age. Health providers have no alternative but to accommodate more rigorous accountability standards in which the quality of care as well as health services' costs are visible.

Adapting to this new consumer-driven environment will test the ability of physicians to forsake traditional authoritarian habits for more collaborative approaches in dealing with patients. The ability of physicians to listen and communicate clearly, together with educational and counseling skills, now ranks alongside medical and surgical skills in importance.

In brief, physicians and hospitals will have to pay more attention to what consumers want and need and, in so doing, restructure health care services that currently are oriented more for the convenience of providers than for the people they serve. Generational differences being what they are, young physicians will have less difficulty in adapting than will their older counterparts whose bedside manner was formed at a time when medical information was considered too esoteric to be grasped by other than health professionals. (For a discussion of new constraints on clinical autonomy and changes in the physician–patient relationship, see Mechanic 2000.)

The consumer health movement signals, among other changes, an end to practices requiring patients to travel to different sites for multiple medical procedures that can be more conveniently rendered seamlessly in a single setting that features easy access and comfortable amenities. Health providers have already begun to move in this direction, but as pointed out by Herzlinger (2007), they still have a long way to go. In the interest both of quality of care as well as cost reduction, she points to the need for restructuring health care to provide disease-specific, one-stop integrated care.

Cost Sharing Revisited

Curbing the inflationary spending that stems from the popular, but misconceived, mindset that health care is a free good when paid for by a third party is one of the more difficult challenges elected officials face. Whatever they do is bound to be unpopular with voters. Inaction, in the hope that the problem will diminish or go away, is unrealistic given the currently unsustainable rate increase in health spending.

So long as national health insurance or single-payer coverage are conceived as vehicles for eliminating the influence of price in the allocation of health services, their adoption will only make matters worse.

Free care is a stimulus for insatiable demand, contrary to what once was thought logical. The gap between what people want and what the system can provide widens with advances in economic development. The pursuit of health, when expressed as a state of total physical, emotional, and mental well-being and not the mere absence of disease, as promulgated by the World Health Organization, is a formula for endless expansion of the boundaries of health care (Battistella 1986: 55–70).

The abuse of generous sick pay and disability benefits in some European welfare state countries is informative in this regard. In Sweden, these payments consume 8 percent of the government's budget or 4 percent of the country's GDP. Swedes, according to the World Health Organization, are among the healthiest people in the world. Yet some 13 percent of working-age Swedes live on some type of disability benefit. During recent World Cup soccer finals sick leave among Swedish men rose by 55 percent (Walker 2007: A1). Disability is also on the rise in Canada, Ireland, the Netherlands, and the United Kingdom despite the lack of any indication that people's health has declined. This suggests that the more people are compensated for complaints like mental and physical stress or bad backs, the more such problems are reported (Finfacts 2007). Health-related job absenteeism among public-sector workers in Italy is considered a plague. In 2005, state employees took an average of eighteen days sick leave. In the health service the figure was almost six weeks (*The Economist* 2008: 52). In comparison, workers in the United States average five sick days a year (Finfacts Ireland).

Well-intentioned, overly generous benefits and the perception of health care as a free good not only contributes to wasteful spending and overconsumption but furthers public indifference to health provider charges and billing practices. This, together with the strong bonds of the physician–patient relationship, creates a politically powerful public-provider coalition for unrestrained spending that makes it hard for elected officials to control—if for no other reason than their dependence on voter favor for job security. Efforts to tame health care will remain an arduous uphill struggle so long as the patient–physician coalition remains intact. It stimulates demand for reimbursement for a constantly expanding array of marginally efficacious services that, like many forms of alternative medicine, cosmetic treatments, and performance-enhancing drugs, stretches the definition of what is medically necessary and appropriate (Mechanic 2006: 39–50; National Council against Health Fraud 2002).

The experiences of Switzerland and England are instructive in this regard. In both countries, expanding government outlays for popular but unproved complementary and alternative medical therapies have sparked cries for investigations into the size and merit of such spending (BMC Health Services Research 2009; Times Online 2006). Constraining voters' penchant for an endless array of services of dubious efficacy is impossible when health care is perceived to be free. Transforming the public from inflation enablers to inflation fighters, while difficult, is an objective that lends itself to a market-oriented solution.

Cost sharing merits consideration given the public's dislike of bureaucratic-style rationing and restrictions on freedom of choice. As demonstrated by the Rand Corporation many years ago and subsequently affirmed by others, first-dollar coverage creates a perverse incentive for overconsumption that significantly declines when consumers are individually responsible to pay a share of the cost. However, the amount has to be large enough to get their attention before it can make a difference. Various levels of co-insurance payments were applied in the Rand study, and total out-of-pocket expenditures were capped so as to not exceed 15 percent of a participant's disposable income. Utilization was found to be directly related to the amount of cost sharing that applied only to outpatient services. Because of the volume of unnecessary and ineffective care, health status generally was unaffected.

This and other studies nevertheless arouse worries that a decline in use of preventive services among low-income children could have adverse future effects that do not show up in the short term. Cost-related under-use of prescription drugs by low-income adults, particularly the chronically ill, raises additional concerns (Gruber 2006). Although significant, these potential limitations do not rule out the use of cost sharing for instilling cost-conscious behavior. Any deleterious effects can be successfully moderated, if not overcome, with the aid of incentives designed to elicit desired behaviors, for example, earmarked preventive care vouchers, capping out-of-pocket payments as a percentage of disposable income, and the use of sliding scale premium subsidies for the low-income uninsured.

Through the selective use of these and other nudge factors it is possible for the government to increase compliance with desirable behaviors. (For an explanation of how the science of choice can be applied to achieve public policy objectives, see Thaler and Sunstein 2008.) Imaginative use of financial incentives by government is an example of where partnership prevails, for whereas markets excel in promoting efficiency, government excels in dealing with equity issues. Counterbalance is the essential element for sound-functioning public–private collaboration.

The danger of deterring access to care for the serious illness is considerably lessened by concentrating cost sharing at the primary care level where most of the utilization that occurs is for conditions that are self-limiting and non–life threatening. The most common reasons people seek primary care are uncomplicated—for example, general physical examination, cough, hypertension, sore throat, and well baby examination (Williams and Torrens 2008: 163–67). Redirecting health insurance on major medical expenses further makes premiums more affordable and does more to safeguard the financial security of households by focusing coverage on serious illness and large-sized medical expenses. In summation, redirecting health insurance from first-dollar coverage to catastrophic coverage is fundamental to practical cost containment.

Uninsured Problem: Extent of True Need

As the nation falls into deeper recession the size of the uninsured population can be expected to increase beyond the present level of 16 percent. Just how much depends on the scale and duration of unemployment as employers eliminate jobs to cut costs and bankruptcies rise. However, for every one percentage point rise in the unemployment rate, the number of uninsured, according to the Kaiser Family foundation, will grow by 1.1 million (Gruber 2002).

Ideally this problem calls for a comprehensive approach but the severity of the strains on the federal budget suggests that an incremental approach may be a more financially prudent choice. Moreover the fact that the uninsured, contrary to popular perception, are not a homogeneous group provides an opportunity for enlisting the private sector to disaggregate the problem and minimize the demands on public financing.

A big and politically controversial component of the uninsured problem involves the government's failure to solve illegal immigration. Of the immigrants entering the country more than half of them are illegal. For the most part they are poorly educated and are employed by low-wage firms that do not provide health benefits or work off the books when performing menial jobs. Thus they are more than twice as likely as persons in native households to be uninsured. Since 1990 nearly 75 percent of the increase in the number of uninsured consists of immigrants and their US born children (Fronstin 2008; Knight 2000; Appleby 2000).

Not all the uninsured are poor. A large number of them have sufficient income to purchase insurance but for various reasons elect not to purchase it (Benko 2003: 8–9, 16). Middle- and high-income families comprise the fastest growing segment of the uninsured population. About 10 percent of households earning more than $50,000 are uninsured. Surprisingly, many high-income Hispanics are found in this category. A cultural unfamiliarity with health insurance leads some of them to forgo insurance even when they can afford it (Fronstin 2007). One-fifth of the uninsured have incomes that are 300 percent or more above the poverty line; and 17 percent have incomes 200 to 299 percent above the poverty line.

Healthy young adults for whom consciousness of health risks is low and whose priorities lie elsewhere comprise another large group. Close to one-third of persons in the 18 to 34 age category are uninsured compared to 14 percent of persons aged 45 to 64. (Herrick 2005). To the extent feasible, it is beneficial to include younger members who can afford coverage into insurance pools. Broadening the pool helps make insurance more affordable for older persons, since the younger group members are healthier and less likely to incur major medical bills.

Many people go without insurance for short periods as they move from one job to another. For this group the problem is largely self-correcting. Nearly two-fifths of the uninsured remain without coverage for periods of four months or less. Only one-third of minority groups experience hard-core uninsurance lasting a year or more (Fronstin 2001).

Persons aged 45 to 64 comprise another fast-growing group among the uninsured. Loss of employment-based coverage from corporate downsizing and layoffs recently has gone beyond blue-collar workers to include white-collar managerial and professional workers (Herrick 2005). An unknown but nevertheless significant number of displaced high-income workers who can afford to purchase individual coverage are choosing not to in order to put their money into starting up a business or some other purpose. The fact that among the uninsured there is a pool of individuals who can purchase insurance either entirely on their own or with the help of public subsidies pegged to income constitutes the rationale, of course, behind proposals that require individuals to buy health insurance.

Regardless of the complex reasons and motivations underlying the uninsured problem, creative financial incentives for the non-poor and sliding scale subsidies for low-income persons would do much to shrink the size of the problem. It is estimated that as many as 20 percent of the uninsured can afford coverage but chose not to purchase it (Dubay, Holahan, and Cook 2006). Involving market forces to limit the strains on government financing is a concept that has evolved from a formerly one-sided association with right wing political ideology to encompass broader legitimacy. It is now apparent that solving the un-insurance problem or implementing universal coverage cannot be done without at the same time adding to the government's budget woes or stifling economic recovery.

Recognition of the necessity for trade-offs is broadening. In the 2008 presidential election both major candidates for the Democratic nomination committed to a private–public partnership concept. Al-though it departs from the Democratic Party's orthodox commitment to taxpayer-financed national health insurance, the idea of private–public collaboration has subsequently been incorporated in the Obama administration's health reform agenda. While factional differences re-main strong in both parties, centrists have rallied around the partner-ship concept. Yet, despite bipartisan agreement on including the private sector in health reform, there is disagreement on how best to do it. In contrast to centrist Democrats who lean toward mandatory purchase and sliding-scale subsidies, Republican centrists are predisposed to en-dorse tax incentives.

However, the rise of pragmatism within the Washington political es-tablishment in dealing with costly health reforms overshadows these ideological disputes and represents a significant turning point in health policy. It is interesting in this regard that, as described later, a number of countries that subscribe to tax-funded health care systems are add-ing market-based competition to spread the burden of financing and encourage efficiencies (PriceWaterhouseCoopers 2009).

Health Care Consumer-Good Status Reconsidered

Policy positions rejecting market competition in health care need to be reconsidered in much the same way as does the rejection of the consumer role. Dismissal of market competition is based on the identi-fication of encumbrances described a half century ago in a highly influ-ential scholarly article that to this day shapes health policy deliberations (Arrow 1963). Within the community of politically liberal reformers it provides a continuing justification for opposing the extension of market principles to health care (Richmond and Fein 2005). It is deeply encoded in their belief system. Needless to say, much has changed with the passage of time. Denials to the contrary, health care today bears many of the features of a consumer good and a considerable amount of utilization is subject to market competition.

Many of the old encumbrances are gone; legal and ethical prohibitions against advertising for patients disappeared decades ago, as have controls granting exclusive powers to allopathic physicians (MDs) for the diagnosis and treatment of illness. Hospitals and physicians now compete openly for patients, and nurse practitioners, together with chiropractors and other nontraditional practitioners, have become increasingly important sources of health care. The expanding role of non-MD health providers owes much to actions taken by state and federal governments that made these providers eligible for reimbursement from health insurers.

Other contributing factors include a shortage of primary care physicians and a public reaction against the cost of orthodox medicine, which moreover is often criticized for being overly specialized and neglectful of the benefits of holistic treatment methods. This is manifested in the growing market for alternative complementary health services. Another important change is that patients actively seek and have better access to reliable medical information. While not eliminated, the one-sided advantage in knowledge possessed by physicians has, as mentioned above, diminished markedly due to the dissemination of medical information in the mass media and greater disclosure of medical prices and quality of care information—all of which is quickly found on the Internet (US Dept of Health and Human Services 2009; National Conference of State Legislatures 2009; HealthGrades 2009; Consumer Reports 2009).

Transparency of previously hard to acquire information in combination with higher educational levels within the general population enables patients to assume more of a partnership role in clinical decision-making and to make independent health care decisions. The combined effect of this new competitive environment is that individuals have more choices than ever before and are better informed than ever before.

The prevalence of market competition in health care today is plain to see in the proliferation of advertisements and marketing strategies in which providers proclaim the excellence of their services in one or more clinical areas (obstetrics, orthopedics, neurology, cancer, heart

disease, stroke, etc.) often based on the findings of studies and evalua-
tions in which their performance is compared with rivals. Competition
is also apparent in the vast sums hospitals and physician groups invest
in improving patient amenities. Another manifestation, while still in
an early stage, is the growing responsiveness of individuals to comparative price and quality information in their choice of provider for
voluntary procedures.

Market competition, something that was previously frowned upon
as unprofessional and unethical, is now commonplace. This is largely
a consequence of federal legislation enacted in the early 1980s to save
money in the Medicare program by changing the way it paid hospitals.
Whether unintended or not the new payment system gave hospitals an
incentive to compete against one another for market share and survival.
While it has done much to stimulate the horizontal and vertical integration of hospitals, competition to date has been misdirected.

The incentives are counterproductive from a social standpoint. They
discourage insurers from enrolling sick individuals and promote ethically questionable billing practices, while discouraging hospitals and
physicians from referring patients to other providers who are more
qualified. The incentives also penalize physicians for spending more
time with patients and encourage hospitals to discharge patients pre-
maturely so that they benefit financially if problems occur and patients
are readmitted. Possibly worse yet, payment does not differentiate between good and inferior care. They both get paid the same.

As pointed out by Porter and Teisberg (2004), competition needs to
be restructured in order to focus on the value of care provided rather
than on the volume of care and to stimulate improvements in efficiency
and quality for which providers currently are not financially rewarded.
In brief, the aim should be to focus competition on specific diseases and
conditions where the largest differences in cost and quality are found,
and to promote cost effectiveness, reduce medical errors, and facilitate
innovation (Porter and Teisberg 2004).

Value-focused competition is not a panacea; it nevertheless is prefer-
able to a single-payer solution. Although a single-payer system would
end the socially dysfunctional selective health insurance enrollment
practices, it would perpetuate the negative incentives of competition.
By shifting power to government, single-payer health care subjects
decision-making to greater political interference and fosters temptations
to save money by shifting costs to other parties (providers, patients, and
employers), limiting patients' access to costly technologies and slowing

the diffusion of innovation. Fortunately, the path of health reform is not proceeding in this direction (Porter and Teisberg 2004).

The net effect of ongoing changes is that much of health care is migrating toward a typical market environment in which more health care fits the definition of a consumer good. Increasingly individuals know the price of what they are buying and have enough information to judge the quality of their purchase, resulting in their ability to make rational choices. This applies especially to routine medical needs at the primary care level and many elective surgical procedures where utilization is discretionary; that is to say, initiated by the individual and not a matter of medical necessity.

Although subject to differing opinions as to what is discretionary and what is necessary, such spending possibly accounts for a third or more of all health spending. This is not an unreasonable estimate. An earlier one made by Pauly (1988) set the amount at roughly 25 percent. His estimate, however, was made in the late 1980s when there was a paucity of transparent price and quality data and when the scope of elective medical procedures was far more limited than those available today. Nor was there, at the time, much information on the use of fast-growing alternative and complementary medical services that people pay for privately. Furthermore health savings accounts were nonexistent. When these two markets are combined, the total amount of out-of-pocket spending approximates over $110 billion (Eisenberg et al. 1998; PBS 2003; American Health Insurance Plans 2009).

An additional $10 to $30 billion is spent annually on cosmetic and lasik surgery (American Society of Plastic Surgeons 2008, 2009). Consumers encounter little difficulty in finding a package price covering all aspects of these procedures and often can make informed choices because providers compete aggressively on price and quality. Prescription drugs is another area where many people are paying out of pocket and shop around for the best prices among competing pharmacies. Some pharmacies are now found in retail stores like Wal-Mart and grocery chains that use prescription drugs as loss leaders to bring in customers.

Yet additional billions are spent by Americans who go overseas for their health care. By the year 2017 this market alone may total $30 billion to $75 billion. According to a recent analysis of medical tourism, more than 750,000 Americans sought less expensive care abroad in 2007, and their number is projected to grow to six million by 2010. Moreover the number of retail primary care clinics is experiencing rapid growth. Their numbers have grown from 250 clinics in 2006 to more than 800 in 2007. (For a description of how retail clinics function, see Turner 2007: A17.)

The effect of all these and related developments—such as employment-based flexible spending accounts, health reimbursement accounts, and retail clinics—is producing a shift away from conventional models of health service delivery to a consumer-centric system of care where price, quality, and service delivery are foremost in importance (Deloitte Center for Health Solutions 2008). The fact that so many hospitals and physicians are resorting to complementary alternative therapies to supplement their income inadvertently is legitimizing the concept of consumer-driven care.

To sum up, individuals' dependence on physicians in health care decision-making has declined as they have become better educated and more knowledgeable about the treatment alternatives available to them. Such knowledge today is much better than in the past, and thanks to information age technologies, and increased price and quality transparency, it is getting better all the time. Boulding (1981) makes a distinction between demand and need that is useful in this regard. Demand implies that individuals possess decision-making autonomy and full knowledge of the available alternatives along with an ability to make informed choices. Need implies the opposite and dependency on expert authority, such as physicians, in making choices.

Growth in the scope of demand coincides conveniently with the trend whereby conventional insurance is beginning to concentrate more on major or catastrophic illness. This union communicates louder than words the changing marketplace for health care. Surely dispassionate analysis is warranted of how co-payments and other forms of out-of-pocket charges can, as urged by Newhouse (2004), be constructively used to reduce nonessential health spending and ameliorate the burden on employer and government financing.

4 Contemporary Realities

National health insurance is an idea whose time has passed. The changes now occurring in employee retirement and health benefits, coupled with the strain of financing similar benefits at all government levels, send a clear signal that the goal of taxpayer-financed universal coverage is unachievable. The visionary principles that have shaped popular conceptualizations of national health insurance remain detached from new realities.

Health care is far more sophisticated and costly than it was at the time the concept of national health insurance was first formulated at the end of the nineteenth century. What was easily affordable then is becoming less so now. Medicine is more effective today, but the cost is increasingly difficult to absorb, to the point where existing arrangements for financing are being pushed to the edge of collapse. Clearly, the old model of health care financing is failing and a new model is required. Although the composition of a new model is in dispute, one thing should be clear: the magnitude of the nation's economic problems impacting both the private and public sectors dictates that any plan for achieving universal coverage be fiscally responsible. Both the private and public sectors are heavily invested in providing health insurance coverage, and both are grappling with serious economic issues.

Employers are under heavy pressure to modify their post–World War II role as the main provider of health insurance, not only because the affordability of offering coverage to employees varies with fluctuations in the business cycle but also because of the high legacy cost they shoulder in providing pension and health benefits for an aging labor force. Large corporations engaged in global markets face an additional problem when competing for business against lower labor cost foreign rivals for whom employee health insurance is not part of their cost of production. In countries where health care is funded out of general revenues, it functions as a tax on profits rather than adding to production costs. Exporters in these countries enjoy an important advantage over American competitors for which heath care financing adds payroll costs (Lowenstein 2008).

In the politics of health reform, the problems besetting American business has become a compelling justification for a government solution among proponents of national health insurance who otherwise have not been noted for harboring pro-business views (e.g., Locke 2009: A13). Supplementing this professed desire to bail out business are claims that postponing national health insurance just because an economy is in recession is analogous to putting a starving person on a diet. During a downturn an economy needs a stimulus, and health spending has a powerful impact in terms of job creation and consumer spending. The traditional message that national health insurance is a moral imperative has been repackaged to read that now it has become a matter of economic necessity (Pipes 2009). Whether sincere or expedient, such justifications nevertheless remain indifferent to the nation's increasing indebtedness and the multigenerational financial burden contained in the size of the governments unfunded future liabilities for entitlement programs.

Federal Deficit Predicament

Deficit spending to finance important national priorities has increased the size of the national debt to such an extent as to jeopardize the government's creditworthiness. The government must balance its spending to match revenues sooner rather than later, since delay will add to the complexity and cost of a solution.

Government expenditures have exceeded revenues in thirty-two out of the last thirty-six years (Bittle and Johnson 2008). Over the next twenty years, annual deficits between seven to 9 percent are forecasted largely because of a surge in entitlement spending from a doubling in the number of elderly qualifying for Medicare and Social Security. According to standard macroeconomic management guidelines developed in the European Union, any deficit level over 3 percent is considered fiscally imprudent. It is highly unlikely that the United States will be able to comply with this norm any time soon.

Deficit management has taken on a new sense of urgency because of the vast outlays expended on programs for combating economic recessions and reviving economic growth. Such spending, together with a weaker economy and past policy choices, caused the 2009 deficit to soar to its highest level at any time since the Second World War. Following a sharp jump into the double-digit range from a stable base of 3 percent, deficits are expected to bottom out in 2013 as a share of the economy and remain in the 5 to 6 percent range for the reminder of the decade. In nominal dollar terms, this translates into annual budget shortfalls of close to $120 trillion.

This is a best-case ten-year scenario, based on assumptions of a full economic recovery and that no new tax or spending policies are enacted during the period. Most important, it excludes a major increase in government-financed health care. It also assumes that Medicare expenditures are restrained by imposing a more than 20 percent reduction in payments to physicians—which is unlikely given the Congress's history of disregarding previously imposed limits (Auberbach and Gale 2009).

As the government has had to borrow more, it has becoming increasingly dependent on foreign lenders. Foreign governments now hold approximately 50 percent of US federal government treasury bonds (Hodges 2009). In as much as this has the potential to limit the government's flexibility in managing the economy, it is a troublesome development. If deficit spending continues unabated along with the amount of national debt, foreign creditors may seek to protect the value of their holdings. They may insist that the US government reduce spending, raise taxes, or pay a higher rate of interest on debt securities to keep foreign lenders from switching their money to sounder investments. In such an event the fallout would have severe domestic political as well as economic consequences. Briefly put, the government risks forfeiting control of the domestic economy to foreign parties, some of who are potential enemies of the United States.

Dependence on foreign creditors also diverts consumer purchasing power out of the country. Debt service payments help feed foreign employment at the expense of domestic employment. Insofar as borrowing is used to sustain short-term indulgences to the neglect of long-term investments, the interest obligations accumulate moreover without creating the wealth needed for paying off the debt (Lewis 2007: 181).

Even if all the debt were held domestically, vast increases in federal spending set the stage for an outbreak of punitively high inflation unless subsequent control measures are taken to slow the economy. The percentage of the federal budget dedicated to debt payment will likely grow substantially beyond the present single-digit level of 9 percent, thereby curtailing leeway for discretionary spending—particularly when combined with growth in fixed entitlement payments for an increasingly aging population. Debt service together with Social Security, Medicare, and Medicaid already account for around 55 percent of the federal budget (Bittle and Johnson 2008).

In paying off the debt, the government also must choose whether to raise taxes or to reduce its fiscal burden through inflationary means. All the debt management options contain disruptive side effects for the economy that challenge the resolve of elected officials to embrace the correct but politically controversial measures. Tax increases risk discouraging investments in job and wealth creation, thereby prolonging unemployment and economic recessions. Inflation may similarly discourage productive investment while eroding the financial security of retirees with fixed incomes (*The Economist* 2009).

Although serious in its own right, the problem raised by the accumulation of debt in recent years is compounded enormously by the size of unfunded future liabilities for Social Security, Medicare, and Medicaid that, depending on how measured, exceeds $40 trillion—a sum more than three times the nation's GDP. Spending for these entitlements is destined to increase in coming years as the large baby boomer cohort passes through the retirement life-cycle stage (Council of Economic Advisors 2009).

Medicare expenditures will grow much faster than Social Security. While increases in the eligible population will affect both funds equally, annual health care spending is expected to rise twice as fast because of continuing medical innovation that extends life expectancy, and greater utilization of more expensive treatments. Medicare also will be pressed to expand the goods and services it covers (Council of Economic Advisors 2009). Already there is considerable political pressure to fill benefit gaps in Medicare's prescription drug component. Voters can be expected to press for still more expanded coverage such as dental, vision correction, long-term care, and complementary alternative medical treatments. Politicians seeking office or job security will be only too happy to oblige.

The history of the Medicare Part B premium is indicative. When first enacted, the program's cost was shared equally by the elderly and the federal government. Since then the share of the program financed from premiums paid by the elderly has declined to 25 percent and the amount paid from general revenues has grown to 75 percent (ElderWeb 2009).

Ironically, the way the government handles revenues from payroll taxes dedicated to these two programs is used to conceal the actual size of the federal deficit. Money collected that is intended as entitlement benefit payments are not directly deposited into their respective trust funds. Rather, IOUs are deposited and Congress spends the money for other purposes, thereby provoking the crack that these funds are a fiscal oxymoron (Peterson 2004).

The federal deficit would be much larger than reported if, as a result of political maneuvering and manipulation of accounting practices, surpluses in the Social Security and Medicare trust funds were not diverted from their stated purpose. In 2008, for example, the real deficit was twice as large as reported (Bittle and Johnson 2008). While under present government accounting rules more money is flowing in than is being paid out for both programs, the outgoing payments soon will exceed income.

Not including interest payments owed on governmental IOUs, Medicare expenditures will exceed incoming revenues starting in 2010, and Social Security will follow in 2017. At that time these programs will start to exert pressure on the rest of the budget. The government will have to cover expenditures by borrowing, funneling money away from other programs, or increasing taxes. Voters are generally unaware of this impending predicament. With few exceptions, elected officials are shy about publicizing this issue, possibly because it requires admitting to the public that the government has made more promises than it can keep (Brookings Heritage Fiscal Seminar 2008).

Congressional reporting based on the government's accounting method distorts the programs' weak financial condition by claiming that the trust funds will not run out of money until a more distant date—2019 in the case of Medicare and 2041 for Social Security—thereby misleading the public as to their fiscal soundness. More recently the expiration dates have been moved up to 2017 and 2037, respectively. When the Social Security trust fund becomes fully exhausted by the creative accounting method now in use, receipts will be sufficient to pay only about 75 percent of promised benefits (Social Security Administration 2009).

Spending for Social Security, Medicare, and Medicaid weigh heavily on the economy. In 2008 spending on these programs amounted to over 8 percent of GDP. If nothing is done, these programs will account for over 10 percent of GDP in 2020 and around 15 percent of GDP by 2040. By 2080 the amount will total nearly 20 percent of GDP. Health spending effects will be especially serious. Government health spending presently constitutes around two-fifths of total health spending, which in turn accounts for one-sixth of the economy. Given its massive size, what happens in the health sector inevitably exerts major repercussions elsewhere in the economy.

The federal budget already is noticeably squeezed by Social Security, Medicare, and Medicaid, and these expenditures are expected to grow. Excluding interest outlays, they now account for close to 45 percent of the federal budget. By 2018 these programs alone may consume as much as three-fifths of the government's budget. The current situation is serious enough. When entitlement spending is combined with other fixed obligations, only 38 percent of the federal budget remains available for discretionary spending. Worse yet, of this amount over half deals with security programs—defense, homeland security, and the war on terror—that in today's international environment are hard to cut. So the actual amount of discretionary latitude in the budget may be as low as 19 percent (*A Citizen's Guide to the 2008 Financial Report of the United States Government*. The Federal Government's Financial Health. http://www.gao.gov/financial/citizensguide2008.pdf).

As the baby boomer generation ages and the full force of this demographic time bomb is felt, future growth in entitlement programs will further limit discretionary spending unless something is done to modify them or federal revenues are substantially increased (Austin 2008). Health care, for reasons cited above, is by far the most serious problem. Over the long term, rising health care costs, according to the Congressional Budget Office, represent the single biggest challenge to balancing the federal budget (Elmendorf 2009).

Precarious State Government Finances

State governments are in an even worse position. They are exposed earlier to the negative effects of economic downturns than the federal government and take longer to recover. Periods of high unemployment increase dependence of low-income populations on social support programs like unemployment benefits, food stamps, and especially Medicaid. This dependence on social support programs happens at the very time when the states are least able to afford paying for them because of balanced budget requirements that call for decreased spending. Although tax increases have been used to finance spending shortfalls, it is infeasible to raise taxes during a recession: tax increases on communities and business make an economic downturn more severe (National Governors' Association 2008).

Medicaid is the largest and fastest growing component of state budgets. It accounts for over 20 percent of overall state spending. As more individuals lose job-based health coverage because employers reduce or eliminate health benefits, lay off workers, or go out of business, Medicaid eligibility and enrollment rises. When this occurs in the midst of an economic recession, it is bad social policy to reduce benefits or eligibility no matter how much pressure there is to reduce spending. Nevertheless, in the last few years forty-five states have cut benefits not mandated by federal law, and Tennessee and Texas removed large numbers of adults and children from their Medicaid rolls due to pressures to cut costs (Emanuel 2008: 23–24). In the best of all worlds, such changes are made during periods of low unemployment and robust economic growth.

The percentage of state budgets going to health spending is significantly higher than that attributed to Medicaid. The cost of other health programs, among which are public health functions and employee health benefits, is a big factor. Altogether, in 2005, health spending comprised approximately one-third of all state spending (Milbank Memorial Fund and National Association of State Budget Officers 2005). Today, the fiscal stress states encounter in fulfilling health spending demands has intensified due to new accounting rules that went into effect in 2008. The standards devised by the Government Accounting Standards Board (GASB statement 45) now require state governments to quantify and report the size of unfunded health liabilities provided to retired government employees. Local government must adhere to the same reporting requirement.

Combining the two levels of government, total liabilities amount to $1.4 trillion (Edwards and Gokhale 2006). Thus many governmental units are debating how to fund their health spending obligation and minimize the impact on their tax rates (Berman and Keating 2006). To be sure, health spending will impair the credit rating of many state and local governments and raise their borrowing costs. Other consequences may follow.

When a similar requirement was imposed on the private sector in the early 1990s, it precipitated major reductions in the scope and continuation of retiree health benefits. It also gave employers an incentive to reduce the number of older workers, through downsizing and early buyout programs, and replace them with younger workers. These events contributed to an increase in the number of low-income retirees under age 65 needing Medicaid assistance; likewise there was an increase in the number of Medicare enrollees who required assistance and, because of greater exposure to health care costs, had become unable to meet the program's deductible and co-insurance requirements.

Pressures exerted on the states to spend more on health care are therefore likely to outweigh those on the federal government. Medicaid annual expenditures already surpass those for Medicare, and are forecast to grow by close to 8 percent yearly over the next decade. This rate has alarmed many state officials. There is a fear that Medicaid will bankrupt every state in the nation unless spending can be brought under control (Pew Center on the States 2006). While the forces responsible for future health spending growth affect both Medicaid and Medicare equally, population aging will exert its impact more severely on the states.

The states, of course, have a much bigger role in financing long-term care, and long-term care represents a much bigger share of the Medicaid budget than is the case for Medicare. Although not intended when originally conceived, Medicaid has evolved into a long-term care program. Medicaid spends two and one half times more on long-term care than does Medicare. Medicaid accounts for roughly 50 percent of all long-term spending (Georgetown University Health Policy Institute 2007). More important, long-term care recipients consume a higher share of Medicaid spending—35 percent on average—than any other recipient group. Spending for this group is destined to grow as the number of elderly increase and more of them enter the life-cycle phase (post 80 years of age) where need for long-term support accelerates.

Liberal eligibility criteria will also contribute to more Medicaid spending. The elderly are not required to be poor in the same way that other Medicaid applicants are. They can easily retain unlimited assets, while qualifying so long as the assets are held in an exempt form and they have high enough medical expenses. The program permits generous exemptions for a residence, family business, and spousal assets. Additionally it is fairly easy to safeguard estate holdings by transferring them to heirs or in a sheltered trust. All that is required is some advance planning and the assistance of one of the many lawyers specializing in such matters (Moses 2005).

Demographic Transition: An Aging Population

In large part the challenges confronting policy makers over the next three decades stem from an impending change in the nation's population structure. The nation is rapidly graying. The number of retirees is growing at the same time that the working-age population is declining. A little more than 16 percent of Americans are now 65 or older, but this soon will change dramatically. The number of elderly will rise to 20 percent in 2020 and 25 percent in 2030, where it will remain for the foreseeable future. Not only are their numbers increasing but also they are living longer. Unless entitlement programs are restructured, this demographic shift will result in the financial collapse of entitlement programs.

Social Security and the hospital component of Medicare are pay-as-you-go systems whose financing rests on an implicit intergenerational contract in which the young provide for the elderly through payroll deductions in the expectation that the next wave of young persons will do the same for them when they become elderly. This arrangement worked well in the past when there were few elderly and many more working-age persons, but it is about to fall apart.

The ratio of workers to retirees will decline by half in the next two decades, and there is not a lot that can be done about this demographic development. Whereas there were 16 workers for every elderly person in 1950, that number has declined to the present level of 3.3, and will decline yet more to 2.6 in 2020 and to 2.1 in 2030 (Department of Health and Human Services 2008).

Spending on these entitlement programs is scheduled to increase much faster than the general economy in future years. Current and future generations of young people are faced with the prospect of bearing much higher costs or receiving fewer benefits than the elderly now receive. In the absence of changes in eligibility criteria and benefit cuts, maintaining these programs at today's level will require raising the combined payroll tax from its present level of close to 15 percent to 37 percent in 2020 and over 50 percent in 2030.

As punitive as this scenario appears, it actually understates the tax burden on working-age adults. Not included are federal income taxes that will have to go up in order to pay for health benefits financed out of general revenues, such as Medicare physician and prescription benefits and Medicaid. State and local property and income taxes will also see increases. Nor are the tax implications included of servicing the massive federal debt load that future generations will have to shoulder—about which more will be said later (Kotzlikoff and Burns 2004).

Many taxpayers now are exempted from paying income taxes and serious political consideration is being given to increasing their numbers from one-third to two-fifths or more of all income earners. To compensate, others will share a larger portion of the tax burden to the point where savings and investment are discouraged, in which case some alternative to the income tax will have to be found that avoids harming the economy (Styring and Jonas 1999).

Considering the magnitude of unfunded future entitlement obligations and the improbability that an easy way can be found to close the funding gap, the government, as said above, is in a predicament. It has made more promises than it can keep. Even so, this and other economic problems that have befallen the nation do not deter national health insurance supporters from pursuing an ideologically driven agenda that, if enacted, would further jeopardize the nation's economic health.

National Health Insurance: A Utopian Driven Vision

There is a utopian quality to national health insurance that underlies its appeal. It conjures an equalitarian image where individuals enjoy unrestrained freedom of choice to health services that are comprehensive in scope and available to all free of charge. Individuals are emancipated from the worry of getting a job that offers health insurance, and the adequacy and permanence of coverage becomes an obligation of government. Within this idealized world individuals possess an inalienable right to free care that is devoid of class distinctions—everyone is entitled to liberally open-ended health care in accordance with their medical needs.

Market forces are abhorrent in as much as differences in income and wealth engender multi-tiered systems and levels of care that violate the ideal of a single standard for all. Profit-driven decision-making moreover undermines and corrupts health care's essential social purpose (Physicians' Working Group 2003; Angell 2009). In short, it is hard to carry on a conversation with true believers. They see national health insurance as the salvation to the problems of the uninsured and the insured that lack sufficient coverage inasmuch as the values that motivate and direct them are too deeply rooted in ideology to concede a need for practicality.

Supporters of comprehensive government-funded free care are predisposed to ignore any mention of the risks of an accompanying free-good mindset. Experience indicates that individuals would demand more health care than they would if they were paying for it themselves, since it personally costs them little to nothing, and that wants and needs become insatiable when care is believed to be free. Rationing health care moreover is something advocates of government-financed health care innocently assume most Americans would willingly accept in the interest of keeping spending under control. The possibility that government price controls might retard innovation and lead to under-investment in physical plant upkeep and modernization is a matter of insouciant disregard.

New Realities' Impact: Some Government Health Policy Scenarios

New realities impacting on government are pressing it to reassess and revise its role in health care financing. Exactly how this will evolve is hard to predict. Nevertheless, certain trend lines are emerging.

The weight of debt that government must contend with over the next several decades necessitates change. Rather than paying for everyone, public financing is apt to focus more closely on special populations in which eligibility is tested for ability to purchase private insurance, and total federal spending is capped to comply with budgetary exigencies and necessity for cost control imperatives. Chances are high that individuals lacking either employer or government health coverage will be required to purchase private coverage from insurers prohibited from denying coverage or charging higher premiums to high-risk applicants.

In order to maximize private coverage while also moderating expenditures, government will find it necessary to subsidize low-income households on a sliding scale basis or through the granting of tax credits. Private insurers will then have to be protected against losses by compensating them for enrolling high-risk individuals through risk-adjusted premiums or other forms of relief. In this context, interest in the voucher plan available to federal employees, the Federal Employee Health Benefit Plan (FEHBP), will receive more attention in any restructuring of the Medicare and Medicaid programs. Briefly described, individuals select an insurer from a menu of previously screened and approved plans for which their premium cost is subsidized. Although not usually thought of as such, FEHBP, for all practical purposes, functions like a voucher plan.

The government contributes the lesser of 75 percent of the premium of the selected plan or 72 percent of the overall average premium of insurers participating in the program. When individuals select a plan with a premium less than the government's contribution, they keep the difference. Conversely, if they chose a more expensive plan, they pay the difference out of their own pocket. The advantage of a voucher system is that it improves financial planning and control. Unlike retrospective payment systems, it enables budget officials to know spending totals in advance of the fiscal year. Vouchers, if properly designed, can also give participants an incentive to shop for the best value plans.

The magnitude of the government's budgetary and fiscal problems also implies continued experimentation with managed care contracting. The Obama administration has sent a strong signal to this effect by declaring its intent to have HMOs compete for Medicare contracts through a competitive bidding process beginning in 2012 (Kronick 2009). Despite criticism that managed care firms are overcompensated for their services, HMOs have established a record of leadership in launching efficiency and quality improvement methods that were once denounced as overly radical but now are considered mainstream— such as primary care gatekeeping, provider profiling, performance-based compensation, disease management, and the application of cost effectiveness criteria in determining payment levels for medical treatments.

The record of not-for-profit managed care firms is especially note-worthy in this connection, as well as for their diligence in applying preventive health measures. Prepayment plans that feature multispecialty group practice and fully integrated delivery systems, such as modeled after Kaiser and Group Health Cooperative of Puget Sound, have long appealed to reformers as a guide to how health care ought to be restructured (for some examples, see Schneider, Zaslavsky, and Epstein 2006 and Kuttner 1998).

Improvement in efficiency and quality of care is broadly considered a necessary precondition for universal coverage to keep subsequent government spending from growing out of control. The financial incentive to shop for the best and least expensive plan must, however, be substantial enough to have the desired effect. In this regard the FEHBP incentive to do so has been determined to be too small. Such selection does not occur because individuals only save 25 cents on the dollar. To be effective, it is recommended that savings have to be much higher (Diamond 2001).

Practicality suggests that health savings accounts (HSAs) now derided for their partisan association may remain an option if promoted under a less invidious label, such as personal health accounts. Given the constraints on public financing, policy makers are bound to contemplate the possibility of having individuals pay for as much health care as they can afford on their own. Governments in South Africa, Singapore, and China now sponsor HSAs as a means of controlling costs by making individuals more cost conscious, but there is some question about their effectiveness.

Critics contend that because HSAs appeal mainly to young and healthy persons, they raise the cost of insurance for all others inasmuch as the pool of persons remaining in employer-based plans is reduced to sicker and older persons who are more costly to cover. Also the higher cost of providing insurance would induce employers to either shift cost to employees or drop coverage entirely, thereby exacerbating the nation's uninsured problem. Another criticism is that rather than getting individuals to become more prudent health care consumers, HSA financial incentives discourage the use of preventive services and timely initiation of health care following the onset of illness symptoms. As a result, when individuals do seek care, they are sicker, and it costs more to treat them.

HSAs are criticized furthermore for discriminating against low-income persons. Because of the existing tax code, upper income persons benefit far more. Thus someone in the 35 percent tax category saves 35 cents in taxes for each dollar put into an HAS, whereas the tax savings steadily decline and disappear for persons in the lower tax brackets. Also the burden of out-of-pocket requirements is inversely related to income to the disadvantage of low-income persons (Center on Budget and Policy Priorities 2009).

Some of these shortcomings are more easily corrected than others. For instance, special purpose payments such as earmarked vouchers could be designed to promote the use of approved preventive health services, and out-of-pocket payments could be capped as a percentage of net disposable income. However, the remaining unsolved social equity issues appear too formidable to acquire a sufficient consensus for incorporating HSAs within any government-financed health program. They are far more likely to continue to play a role in employer-sponsored health benefit plans. Regardless, they will certainly remain an attractive choice for young and healthy persons seeking affordable individual coverage—especially higher income persons as they benefit most from the tax advantages.

Nevertheless, it is noteworthy that in European health care systems the subject of health savings accounts is receiving some attention as a cost containment option, no matter how implausible in light of their commitment to collective responsibility. That the subject has become worth reviewing speaks to the financial strains on government-funded health care programs posed by an aging population and the cost of new medical treatments. (Thomson 2008).

In the midst of considerable uncertainty, one thing is clear. The government's financial duress signals an end to open-ended fee-for-service reimbursement of physicians and hospitals. One alternative is to pay providers a lump sum for each illness treated using Medicare's hospital prospective payment system as a model. Another approach would relate payment to treatment outcomes. Such improvements in efficiency and quality of care are broadly considered a necessary precondition for whatever form of universal coverage is enacted if subsequent government spending is to be prevented from growing out of control.

Employers' Response to New Realities

Employers likewise are under considerable pressure to modify their role in financing health care. According to a recent survey, employers who offer health benefits do so because they believe it is necessary to recruit and retain workers in a competitive labor market. Most also believe health benefits contribute to worker productivity. However, few believe that it is their role to ensure that employees have coverage. Instead, they prefer to focus on providing access to affordable health plans (Fronstin and Blakely 2008).

Declines in employers' ability to offset higher benefit cost by raising product prices, cutting employee compensation, or reducing payments to shareholders, coupled with annual rates of increase in insurance premiums that exceed the rate of general inflation, create an inducement for small firms to pass more of the cost to employees or discontinue providing health insurance altogether. Those employers that remain committed to retaining coverage will be drawn to more affordable low-cost plans such as the health savings accounts described above. Along with costing less than conventional coverage, these HSAs enable greater predictability and control of health spending inasmuch as they permit employers to fix expenditures in advance of the fiscal year.

Large employers, most of whom are self-insured, are no less interested in obtaining greater predictability and control over their health expenditures. However, because of their superior resources and greater reluctance to reduce or stop offering coverage, vouchers are apt to be a more appealing choice for keeping spending under control. To date, large employers have achieved acceptable success through a variety of measures that, in addition to the savings from self-insuring, include managed care, provider performance monitoring, disease management, and performance-based provider compensation (Galvin 2008).

Still, interest in vouchers can be expected to accelerate if the federal protections enacted in the mid-1970s that have insulated self-insured employers from state regulations continue to erode. Loss of such protection will expose employers operating in multiple states to costly and confusing arrays of state and national regulations that will destabilize and compromise their continued ability to contain health expenditures (Pierron and Fronstin 2008). Increased exposure to the jurisdiction of state courts, in particular, will make it too risky for them to continue direct involvement in efficiency and quality improvement efforts for fear of exposure to medical malpractice litigation and mammoth punitive damage payments. Resorting to vouchers effectively insulates employers from accusations of interfering with the practice of medical charges (Battistella and Burchfield 2000).

Paradoxically, if some public policy changes now contemplated are enacted, they unwittingly may present a low-cost opportunity for employers to get out of the business of providing health insurance in such a way that also insulates them from political criticism. Unless penalty payments for not providing worker coverage contained in mandatory coverage proposals now under consideration are set high enough, they will comprise an open invitation for employers to offload this function to the public sector. To a Machiavelli-minded single-payer partisan, low penalty fees constitute a backdoor strategy for achieving national health insurance. This is an even stronger possibility in the case of mandatory purchase proposals containing a public plan option that, in the guise of expanding choice, would compete with private plans. The government then could use its regulatory, pricing and taxing powers to favor its own plan (e.g., see Carney 2009; Marks 2009).

While large employers are less apt to cease providing health insurance, those with an aging workforce and large retiree population either will follow the example of domestically owned automobile manufacturers and transfer retiree health costs to workers' unions or will seek to have government assume responsibility (e.g., see Stoll 2009). Among the big three domestic automobile manufacturers there are more than two retirees and their surviving spouses for every active employee. General Motors is the worst off. It has a ratio of 4.6 to 1. Retiree health benefits add about $1,500 in health costs to every car produced by GM. This gives its foreign-owned competitors who are spared this expense a big advantage, and it feeds the quip that GM is a health company that makes cars on the side (Perry 2008; Dalmia 2007).

Among firms retaining coverage, cost shifting to employees will persist so long as insurance premiums continue to outpace general inflation. However, conventional cost-shifting tactics (premium charges, deductibles, co-insurance, co-payments, and elimination of family and retiree coverage) either have or soon will reach their limit. At this point employers will be inclined to recognize the incentives inherent in first dollar coverage and shift the focus of health insurance to major medical expenses through means of high-deductible health plans. This is the current trend, and should it fail to work, more employers can be expected to give serious thought to getting out of the business of providing health insurance (Fronstin 2007).

High-deductible plans are grounded in the assumption that individuals can afford to privately pay for most routine health care needs. This returns health insurance to a core insurance principle of providing protection against unwanted and unpredictably large expenditures that endanger household financial security. Conventional health insurance, in comparison, is designed to motivate individuals to make early and frequent use of health care. Inviting the use of health insurance benefits contradicts a fundamental insurance principle.

Many employers are now experimenting with a more sophisticated version of high-deductible health insurance. Employees are given incentives to enroll in some type of consumer-directed health plan such as a tax-free health savings account to which, for purpose of illustration, individuals are permitted to contribute a maximum of $1,500 per year. At the time of this writing around 50 percent of large corporations surveyed have offered a consumer-directed plan and one-fifth of their employees have participated. While the deductibles typically are steep, up to $2,000 or more for an individual and $5,000 for families, many employers, though not required to, make annual contributions to the account, thereby keeping out-of-pocket costs at an affordable level for most individuals.

As a way to discourage wasteful consumption and energize consumer price consciousness when choosing a health provider, money not spent is permitted to accumulate in tax-free investment in much the same way as allowed in defined-contribution pension plans (Watson Wyatt National Business Group on Health 2009). Barring serious misfortune in the first year or two, the money that accumulates in these accounts is more than sufficient to meet most out-of-pocket requirements. Because of the power of tax-free compounding of investments, these accounts have the potential to become a significant retirement nest egg for individuals who remain prudent consumers of basic health services. This is not implausible given the favorable odds individuals have of remaining healthy before reaching retirement age. The viability of these accounts as savings vehicles is supported by findings that less than half of the funds in HAS accounts in 2007 were spent on health care (Zycher 2009).

The innovative aim of health savings accounts is to enlist consumers as partners in cost containment by allowing them to share in any efficiency savings. Shortsighted avoidance of efficacious care by individuals preferring to build savings in their health account is avoidable through the creative use of financial incentives. Toward this end designated vouchers, as described earlier, provide a noncoercive way to nudge consumers into using appropriate preventive health services and follow a healthy lifestyle. The principle behind this approach is to retain the freedom of individuals to make choices but to arrange the choices in a way that increase the probability that they will make the socially desirable choice. Employers, for example, do this when they offer lower health insurance premiums and other rewards to employees who participate in weight control, blood pressure, cholesterol, and smoking withdrawal programs. Also, once health care is initiated, the application of disease management methods provides a way to minimize noncompliance with medical advice, for example, by systematically reminding individuals not to skip prescribed medications and by follow-up physician visits (Battistella and Burchfield 2003).

Summary

The message of this chapter is twofold. National health insurance orthodoxy will have to be rethought to accommodate the unhappy fact that the federal government has already promised more in entitlement benefits than it can deliver without substantially altering the terms of its implied contract with the American public, and the cost to employers of providing first-dollar coverage to their employees is fast reaching a prohibitive level. This predicament, however, does not detract from the imperative for universal health coverage. Rather, it signals the need for greater creativity and practicality in meeting this goal.

New economic and demographic realities furthermore point to a need to reconsider the degree to which insurance ought to shield individuals from health care costs. Increased individual responsibility, scaled to ability to pay, is requisite to devising a program of universal coverage that is fiscally responsible.

5   Popular Misconceptions

From its inception at the beginning of the twentieth century, the history of national health insurance politics in the United States has been a quest for social equity and justice. Because so much of it is advocacy driven, a surprisingly large amount of health reform thinking has fallen under the influence of emotion in which faith and hope prevail over dispassionate analysis and facts. Values derived from theological and philosophical principles play a large part in this reform movement. Although less pronounced and devoid of the emotional intensity found in the politics of national health insurance, faith nevertheless underlies the claims made on behalf of other health reform objectives. A number of misconceptions are unveiled in this chapter and discussed in the context of the aspirations to which they are connected.

First among them is the purported cost savings claimed on behalf of single-payer coverage and belief in bountiful government provided free care. A second misconception centers on the notion that health status and longevity are directly correlated with health spending. A third heralds the advantages of centralized planning and control over decentralized market forces. A fourth misconception is that spending on preventive health services will produce big savings. The idea that universal coverage will eliminate social disparities in health care is another conviction that is grounded more in faith than real world experience. Finally, promulgation of the safety and efficacy of health care stems from a reverential belief in the infallibility of scientific process and the adherence of health professionals to a code of conduct that protects patients from harmful medical treatment.

Single-Payer Coverage Lowers Health Spending

Single payer plans attract the attention of the economy minded as well as dedicated supporters of government-sponsored health care. While unquestionably saving money by eliminating high overhead costs incurred by multiple competing private insurers, the benefits from emulating other countries are oversold (Aaron 2003). When making cross-national comparisons, advocates fail to include differences in accounting practices and adjustments for currency values, and they disregard increases in spending that accompany the removal of financial constraints on health care utilization. Nor do they account for the hidden costs of tax collection and compliance, lobbying, and the administrative burdens shifted on to health providers. Also concealed is the cost of unfunded future entitlement liabilities. Government-financed health systems fail to set money aside to cover future obligations. Expenditures are on a pay-as-you-go basis, on the assumption that the public always remains able and willing to bear whatever tax increases are required.

Regardless of the appropriateness of cross-national comparisons, extending coverage to the presently uninsured population and improving coverage for the underinsured will result in a major spending increase. This is no small matter. Although it is impossible to estimate accurately the cost of a new program before the basics are finalized, a number of health experts believe that the amount of spending required in the decade following enactment of universal coverage will be in the range of $1.5 to $1.7 trillion. This represents an increase of about 4 percent above projected ten-year outlays—a huge amount that raises troublesome questions about the sustainability of universal coverage (Alonzo-Zaldivar 2009; Fox News 2009)

Insofar as individuals receive care for health needs previously forgone, this is to be applauded rather than decried. In point of fact the multiplier effect stemming from the free-good psychology stirred by the possession of health insurance acts as a stimulant for overconsumption. When conjoined with open-ended fee-for-service provider reimbursement, the negative effect is much greater. Besides creating opportunities for providers to raise prices, it allows for medically questionable and unnecessary demands for prescription drugs, diagnostic tests, medical appliances, and costly therapies in place of equally effective less costly alternatives. Expectations and demands also escalate for expanding coverage beyond essential physician and hospital services. As demonstrated by Mechanic (2006), pharmaceutical firms seize opportunities to develop new revenue sources by defining new conditions that fit their products and medical specialists are quick to exploit new diagnostic and treatment methods to generate lucrative income streams (e.g., see Abramson 2005: 149–67).

Mandates imposed on insurers by state legislators for the broadening of benefits beyond basic health services illustrate how politicians contribute to the expansion of what should be covered and treated. Such requirements introduced by state legislators numbered 1800 in 2004 compared to only seven in 1965. Among the many questionable mandates are provider coverage to include chiropractors, podiatrists, optometrists, massage therapists and naturopaths, and such benefits as well-child care, acupuncture, massage therapists, hair prostheses, and performance-enhancing drugs like Viagra (Bunce and Wieske 2004).

If well intentioned, these mandates nevertheless have the unintended consequence of exacerbating the uninsured problem. They not only drive up the cost of health insurance and make it less affordable; they typically preclude insurers from offering innovative low-cost policies that enable some of the uninsured to obtain otherwise unaffordable coverage. Mandated benefits are likely to increase the cost of health insurance by as much as 25 percent. It is estimated moreover that one in four among the uninsured lack coverage because of the cost of state health insurance mandates (National Association of Health Underwriters 2009). If not included at the onset, acquiescence to public pressures for first-dollar coverage compounds the escalation of health spending.

Cost containment is further impaired because of political interference. Politicians, dependent on voter support, eagerly endorse popular demands for more free care and, as occurred in the political backlash against managed care in the 1990s, fail to support unpopular but effective cost restraint initiatives. While this disposition to please is natural to democratic legislatures, the advent of opinion polling and focus groups has made elected officials even more susceptible to popular will and reluctant to exercise fiscal restraint (Kaiser 2009). In this context Congress has a notorious reputation for underestimating the cost of expensive new benefit programs in order to minimize opposition. For example, the 1990 expenditure target it projected for the hospital portion of Medicare was seven times lower than what actually transpired (Hayward and Peterson 1993).

In truth, single-payer health care does have the capability to constrain spending, but it requires the political resolve to impose unpopular measures that US politicians are unlikely to endorse. As discovered in England following enactment of the National Health Service, pressures for increased spending are ceaseless because of ambiguity in the definition of what constitutes sickness and medical need. Sickness, as noted by Cooper (1975), is a relative state that is amenable to almost infinite interpretation by both patients and physicians. Thus the National Health Service, which set out to abolish medical need, failed. Ultimately the only effective way to restrain otherwise uncontainable spending is through command-control rationing. However, even this has its limitations as indicated by the introduction of consumerism and the re-orientation of the National Health Service from a social model to a business model under the auspices of a left of center government historically committed to socialist principles (Pollock 2004).

Health Status and Longevity Are Purchasable

Although the World Health Organization suggests that health care is purchasable and that health care is primarily responsible for improvements in health status and life expectancy experienced throughout the world, even a cursory look at international comparisons indicates that skepticism and qualification are warranted and that the role of health care is overrated (World Health Report 2000). While clearly applicable to poor and emerging economies, the relationship has to be qualified at higher levels of social and economic development where other factors intervene. In the case of infant mortality, factors like income distribution, education, and ethnic and religious composition account for more of the gains than government health spending (Filmer and Pritchett 2004).

Within the community of highly developed countries the contribution of health services to health is, as concluded by Fuchs (1981), very small. Income distribution is a far more significant contributor to longevity and so are such other health indictors as obesity, depression, and teenage pregnancy (Wilkinson and Pickett 2009). The diminishing returns from health spending were recognized by the Canadian government in a highly influential report published in the mid-1970s that placed great emphasis on nonmedical behavioral and environmental determinants (Lalonde 1974).

Gains understandably occur more slowly and diminish following the conquest of major causes of morbidity and mortality linked to poverty and underdevelopment such as infectious diseases, unsafe water and food supplies, unsanitary waste disposal, and malnutrition. Longevity improves rapidly following improvements in maternal and child health and control of communicable diseases, before slowing as living standards progress, birth rates decline, and chronic and degenerative disorders rise. The benefits of spending plateau and returns on spending gradually become smaller as populations age. Not only is the percentage of elderly sharply increasing in industrialized countries but persons over 80 comprise the fastest growing segment of the population.

Since improvements in life expectancy are inversely related to age, any future improvements attributable to health spending will be marginal. Although it seems to indicate otherwise, this is borne out in a recent study by Barr (2006) and Cutler et al. (2006). Between the years 1960 and 2000, life expectancy for newborns increased by close to seven years at a calculated cost of roughly $20,000 each year of life gained over the four-decade-long period. Even though the cost per year of life gained increased to roughly $32,000 in the 1990s, the money spent was still considered to represent good value. However, the value of spending was found to be much smaller for older age groups, and from age 65 and up the costs provided no gain in life expectancy.

While the Cutler study suggests that life expectancy is indeed purchasable, it provides no information on the health status of survivors and the cost of continuing health and social care services. Premature infants and infants with congenital disorders in particular benefited from increased survival rates because of improvements in neonatal health services. However, as discussed earlier, they are often susceptible to other future disabilities and a lifetime need for costly medical and social services. Moreover, in establishing the value of health spending, the study made a questionable inferential leap in assuming that half the gains in life expectancy were due to medical care.

Using life expectancy as a measure of the value of health spending may miss a more important point and misdirect public policy. Within the context of advanced socioeconomic development where life expectancies are starting to push the biological envelope, and the financing of elderly health and social services weighs heavily on society, focusing on whether health services make people more productive, such as treatment of gastric ulcers, cataracts, rheumatoid arthritis, and hearing and orthopedic disorders, may be more advisable. Policies that improve health without affecting life expectancy are key to increases in productivity that ultimately make generous social welfare programs affordable.

Compared to other rich countries, the United States spends twice as much per capita than the next biggest spender, but this does not correlate to the life expectancy results, which by international standards are mediocre. Many other peer countries spend much less and achieve better results on basic health measures while also making health care more widely available and experiencing fewer quality-of-care problems (US Senate Finance Committee 2009). Japan, for example, ranks fifteenth among thirty highly developed countries in health spending but occupies the top spot in life expectancy (Gould 2004). Not only do people in other countries live longer, but, as reported by Daschle (2008), in some instances they also fare better on such indicators as diabetes, arthritis, high blood pressure, and obesity. However, this comparison may be less revealing than it appears.

Public health measures possibly are too broad to reflect health improvements in other areas (Coyne and Hilsenrath 2002: 30–33). Higher spending, for instance, enables a better supply and distribution of technologically intensive services with the result that citizens with serious illnesses have both greater access to medical specialists and better survival rates. In this regard the best survival rates for adults afflicted with certain cancers are found in the United States, and Americans suffering heart disease and stroke obtain higher quality survival time than counterparts elsewhere (Gratzer 2006: 174–78; Cutler 2004: 47–60).

It may also be the case that correlation of health spending to health status is positive but concealed under the inefficiency and waste from the outdated way that health care is financed and delivered in the United States. Gaps in insurance coverage are especially significant in that they keep mainly low-income people from obtaining timely care so that they are much sicker and more expensive to treat when finally seen. The fact that roughly one in six Americans is uninsured is an anomaly to observers from countries where universal coverage is taken for granted. Socioeconomic differences in the distribution of health personnel and facilities further disadvantages poor persons by rendering care less accessible and by exposing them to providers and services that are generally inferior to those found in higher income areas. This is not a problem peculiar to the United States. The supply and distribution of health resources generally is inversely related to medical need and is so prevalent that it has been granted the status of a health care law—the Inverse Need Law (Hart 1971).

Notwithstanding numerous structural and financial deficiencies in US health care, Americans do not appear to be any less healthy than their counterparts in other highly developed countries. To the contrary, when ranked by the prevalence of 35 high-cost medical conditions accounting for close to two-fifths of US health spending, including heart conditions, trauma, cancer, mental health disorders, and diabetes, the United States fared better on 21 medical outcomes than comparable countries such as France, Germany, Italy, Spain, and the United Kingdom (McKinsey Global Institute 2008: 87–89).

Besides deficiencies in the way care is structured and delivered, there are some complications to keep in mind. For example, differences in the definition and reporting of live births distort international comparisons. Another and bigger problem with international comparisons is that they fail to consider the effects of confounding social factors. Population differences in racial and ethnic diversity, family structure, teenage mothers and low birth weight babies, obesity rates, violent crime, employment security, and income inequality are examples of the many things that can mask the positive effect of health spending (Mankiw 2007). US society is far more heterogeneous in its population mix. Wider income disparity among residents, larger numbers of low-income immigrants, and higher rates of job insecurity also differentiate the United States from other industrialized countries that have more homogeneous and healthier populations to start with, some of which has to do with genetic, ethnic, and cultural factors (Garber and Skinner 2008).

Despite confusion in the interpretation of the causes of international differences in health status, the US payment system invites the overuse of costly medical procedures. As much as 30 percent of Medicare spending is due to an overuse of services that could be dispensed with and not have any deleterious effects on health. There is considerable regional variation in illness-specific treatment costs of the elderly without any noticeable difference in quality or outcomes, and the differences far exceed any differences in living costs. For example, it cost 50 percent more to have the same surgical procedure done in a medical center in Boston than in a similar medical center in Minnesota. Likewise treatment costs for particular medical conditions are much higher in Florida and New York than in Utah and Tennessee (Fisher et al. 2003: 288–98).

Much of this overuse is attributable to incentives that have spurred a proliferation of high-technology services to the neglect of primary or basic health care needs. The intensity of care provided in US hospitals is much higher than in other nations. The same is true for rates of cardiac surgery and the availability of costly diagnostic technologies such as magnetic resonance imaging (MRI), computerized axial tomography (CAT) machines, and nuclear particle accelerators (Garber and Skinner 2008). It is not easily determined whether spending will remain the same, decline, or grow if savings from questionable and unnecessary spending is redirected to the uninsured and less costly underused services.

Amid all the ambiguity and confusion, however, the rate of return from spending on health care indisputably declines as a population ages. From a purely investment standpoint, the highest returns are obtained from spending directed at the young. In the final analysis, national prosperity, together with the populations' overall health status, depends on maintaining a judicious relationship between investment and consumption spending. Presently the federal government spends four times more on persons over 64 than it spend on children under the age of 18, raising questions over the implications of such a gap for the nation's future (Edwards and DeHaven 2003).

Moreover, as the elderly population is growing at a faster pace than the rest of the population for decades to come, programs targeted to the elderly will, barring an offsetting increase in revenues, absorb a proportionately larger share of the federal budget so that there will be less money for everything else. A forecast by the Urban Institute indicates the by the year 2050 this will amount to roughly 70 percent of the federal budget (Penner and Steurle 2003).

Recent changes in England's National Health Service underscore the financial imperatives behind trade-offs between consumption and investment in the allocation of public spending on the elderly. For all practical purposes, long-term care no longer is provided to all as a right that is free of charge. Instead, a system of charges has been introduced on an ability-to-pay basis so that only low-income elderly remain eligible for free care (Pollack 2004).

Superiority of Centralized Planning and Control

Although eminently plausible in theory, the results of centralized planning and control rarely perform to expectations. The reasons for this are several. The sheer complexity of real world conditions surpasses the capacity of experts and their analytical models, regardless of how brilliant or sophisticated they are. Health care provides a case in point.

Many of the causes of the steep increase in spending following passage of Medicare and Medicaid alerted federal policy makers to structural shortcomings in health care that if left alone would make spending hard to control and result in wasteful expenditures. At issue were the too many features left from an earlier and simpler health care age that absorbed new money without producing more or better care. Pouring a vast amount of new money into health care was eschewed as tantamount to practicing twentieth-century medicine within a nineteenth-century cottage industry framework.

This concern led the Congress to enact a number of planning initiatives, which in partnership with state governments sought to bring health services in line with modern managerial and corporate practices (Philip and Benjamin 2002: 352–72). Among other objectives, the government sought to reduce costs by imposing controls on the supply of hospital beds, and stimulating the growth of medical group practice plans and not-for-profit health maintenance organizations that provided comprehensive and integrated services for a fixed annual fee (Asron and Schwartz 1984: 3–11). It also sought to raise quality of care standards by reviewing the quality and appropriateness of hospital services provided to Medicare and Medicaid beneficiaries, and by encouraging the concentration of costly complex surgical procedures in high-volume hospitals. By the end of the 1970s the failure of these efforts allowed for the sanctioning of hitherto suspect market principles (Battistella 1972). The result was the proliferation of for-profit corporate hospital chains and for-profit health maintenance organizations.

Reliance on competition has subsequently grown to the point where it has become a primary instrument of choice in efforts to modernize the way health care is structured and delivered. A particularly significant breakthrough occurred when Medicare subjected hospitals to prospective payment in the early 1980s and unleashed incentives that stimulated competition for market share in an industry that had traditionally been sheltered from market forces (Falcone and Hartwig 1997: 135–54). This injection of market initiatives in large part stemmed from frustration within the Congress over the slow pace of progress from centralized planning and control mechanisms.

Prospective payment was a way to spur efficiency and quality improvements by replacing cost-plus fee-for-service hospital reimbursement with a system of fixed payments for each of a large number of specific diagnoses. Hospitals would lose money when their cost of treating a specific condition was more than the government allotment. Conversely, they would make money when their cost of treatment was less. However, unforeseen consequences intervened to thwart this system.

Rather than undertake the arduous and frequently controversial task of requiring physicians to improve their practice methods following the change in reimbursement method, hospitals generally determined it was easier to expand market share through aggressive marketing and advertising, thereby permitting economies of scale and enhanced ability to withstand pressure from HMOs to cut prices. Another consequence of the change in reimbursement was that it stimulated mergers and acquisitions and the formation of multiple hospital systems in order to improve access to capital. Lending institutions regarded hospitals as a bigger credit risk following the loss of Medicare cost-plus reimbursement that on average accounts for 30 percent of hospital revenues (Medicare Payment Advisory Commission 2003).

Efforts to improve the efficiency with which specific medical and surgical procedures are done typically followed the exhaustion of easier revenue enhancing strategies and, for the most part, remains in the early development stage due to the challenge of changing physicians' clinical practice methods. Marketing to prospective patients in competition with other hospitals remains a principal means of assuring sufficient revenue flow. Prior to prospective payment it was considered unprofessional for hospitals to compete against one another for patients. What competition occurred was friendly and in pursuit of prestige. It has since become more of a cutthroat struggle for survival.

It is folly to assume that decision-making by experts is a replacement for conflict and politics. Compliance seldom defers to expertise and objectivity. Studies of regulatory agencies indicate that they soon fall under the influence of the very interests and activities that they are supposed to be controlling and thereby compromise their independence. Special interest groups use regulatory bodies to obtain advantages through regulation that they are unable to achieve in the marketplace. This is the substance of the so-called capture thesis of regulation (Knoll 1974: 25–28). Frequent complaints that the Food and Drug Administration is captive to the pharmaceutical industry provides an example of this practice (Abramson 2005: 85–91). Special interest groups also often have the resources to hire superior legal talent and can hold a regulatory body hostage to lengthy legal delays when objectionable decisions and rules are contested in the courts. When failing to prevent or modify undesirable decisions, special interest groups resort to other means. The success of lobbying as a business attests to this.

Susceptibility to undue political intrusion adds to the limitations of centralized planning. Command of oversight and budgetary appropriations gives politicians considerable advantage in dealing with experts. In deciding whether to side with experts or an important constituency group, politicians choose the latter. They are predisposed to favor those they represent.

A combination of political interference and successful legal challenges were the undoing of state and federal government efforts to curtail costly overlap and duplication of health facilities by requiring a hospital to demonstrate a community need as a condition for obtaining approval from planning agencies to expand their number of beds or purchase costly new technologies. Most studies determined that these controls were ineffectual. Contrary to the intended purpose, these planning agencies were co-opted by existing hospitals to protect themselves from outside competition, the biggest threat of which came from newly emerging publicly traded hospital corporations. (For examples, see Conover and Sloan 1998 and Feldstein 2007.)

Centralized decision-making, under the supervision of elected officials, is moreover impaired by the fact that politicians seldom have comprehensive knowledge of the issues; their role is to represent constituents on a myriad of topics as well as face the innumerable demands of campaigning. Restructuring health care requires a complex solution to a complex problem. There is no easy way to convey to politicians the highly specialized, technical, and financial aspects of health care, as well as clinical content involved. Indeed the danger that partially informed decision-making may unwittingly compound the problem rather than resolve it is omnipresent. The availability of staff helps some, but they too generally lack proper training and experience, or they leave for other career opportunities before benefiting from on-the-job training. Besides, like politicians, staffs are easy prey for lobbyists and other favor seekers.

Even under the best circumstances it is only through pretension alone that Congress can claim to be able to micromanage anything as vast and complicated as health care. In part, this is underscored by the sheer volume and opacity of the 100,000 pages of regulations to be complied with in the Medicare program, (Gratzer 2007: 77). Complexity of regulatory language and voluminous detail is a source of costly differences of interpretation and fraudulent behavior. The difficulty of setting prices for each of the many diagnoses contained in the Medicare prospective payment program provides another example. As noted by Aaron (1996), approximately ten thousand separately defined medical diagnoses exist, many of which are further differentiated by degree of severity and by the presence of complicating patient conditions.

International comparisons certainly show that countries having control of financing spend less on health care. They accomplish this through global budgeting and rationing access to costly services by containing the diffusion of expensive new technologies and the imposition of waiting lists for elective procedures. However, the economies obtained are not an unqualified blessing. The savings often come at the expense of convenience and delays in treatment and follow-up services that feed public grievances and may not meet appropriate care standards. An environment develops in which "everything is perceived to be free but nothing is readily available—a situation reminiscent of health care in the former Soviet Union" (Gratzer 2006: 169; Knaus 1981)

A recent Canadian experience is instructive. The Canadian Supreme Court declared that the government ban on private health insurance was unconstitutional. The ban resulted in treatment delays detrimental to good patient care and was a violation of freedom of choice. Canada is one of the few countries in the world to ban private health insurance providing coverage for items already provided by the government's health plan. The court concluded that the public interest was not served by shielding the public sector from competition. When Canadians are unable to obtain care because they cannot find a physician or have to endure long waits for treatment and follow-up, their situation, in the opinion of some critics, starts to resemble that of uninsured Americans (Geddes 2005; Fraser Institute 2008).

Although private health insurance remains an option in England, delays in securing medical appointments and treatment in its national health service are a long-standing source of professional criticism and public dissatisfaction. In response to these complaints, a traditionally anti-market Labor government was moved to introduce market principles in government-run health services as a way to overcome obstacles to efficiency improvements. Among other changes, formerly excluded for-profit hospitals are now allowed to compete against government hospitals in order to shorten delays in scheduling elective surgical procedures. Reportedly, more than 42,000 persons out of roughly one million on waiting lists for surgical treatment were told recently that they must wait a year for heart, cataract, or joint replacement surgery. The undercapitalization of plant and equipment is another frequent complaint (Cowell 2001; Smith 2005: 173–74). For instance, the English national health service retains many outworn and outmoded facilities, some of whom predate the First World War, because of a history of underfunding (Gaffney et al. 1999). Enlisting the aid of private capital therefore is seen as a way to alleviate shortages of public financing while for-profit competition is meant to stimulate and provoke an otherwise unresponsive health bureaucracy into becoming more efficient.

Popular disenchantment with rationing sparks political demands for government to relax centralized spending controls. In order to preserve budgetary discipline, governments then generally maintain equilibrium by raising taxes and fees. In addition to requiring individuals to pay more out of pocket, parallel private fee-for-service systems are allowed in order to neutralize the opposition of politically sophisticated high-income groups, who insist on a better standard of care than available under government auspices (e.g., see Regional Committee for Europe 2002). Canada has been a notable holdout, though it too is heading in this direction.

Protestations in Canada against moving to a tiered system are somewhat fallacious in as much as individuals financially capable of doing so are able to see physicians on a fee-for-service basis. In many parts of Canada there is growing interest in exploring private-sector solutions for relieving financial pressures on provincial government budgets and delays in treatment and crowding due to government cutbacks (Beltrame 2000). Individuals who can afford it increasingly have access not only to US healthcare providers but also, thanks to the Internet and medical tourism companies, to the global health care market. Although it is not known how many Canadians travel abroad for health care, the possibility of this option is receiving greater media attention as financial pressures on the national and provincial governments contribute to more delays in obtaining health care and frustration within wealthy and middle-class communities deepens (Turner 2007).

Centrally controlled health systems are further susceptible to pressure from powerful health worker unions and professional staff. High salary demands unaccompanied by offsetting productivity and quality improvements are, for example, a principle cause of the British government's solicitation of bids from for-profit entities to provide a competitive challenge to state-run health services. During the 1970s militancy on the part of health staff labor unions was a frequent cause of disruption in patient services. Part of the problem may be that workers are prone to assume that the power of government to print and borrow money is limitless (Seldon 2004; Gorsky 2008).

Market mechanisms are more effective than centralized control and planning mainly because they curtail political interference in decision-making by, as noted earlier, depersonalizing and diffusing responsibility for decisions that inflict pain and discomfort. By granting the parties involved an opportunity to affect their own fate, competition has the effect of restraining political intervention and litigation.

In addition to feeling more personally responsible for outcomes, individuals are disposed to resign themselves to determinations of the proverbial invisible hand if market-based solutions are viewed as reasonably fair.

The practical significance of market competition for expediting otherwise hard to achieve efficiency and quality improvements helps explain why it is finding greater application in health care. This is not to be confused as a triumph of right wing ideology. Rather, it is more appropriately seen as a concession to real world constraints. The difficulty of controlling health expenditures and the anticipated heavier demands for greater spending on entitlement programs and continued medical innovation inevitably pushes policy makers to subordinate ideology to practical necessity in which decisions are based on whether recommended actions are workable and financially responsible. This is occurring in other developed countries as well as in the United States. They too are having to deal with the effects of the high cost of new medical breakthroughs and increased health care utilization due to population aging, which is occurring even at a faster rate than in the United States. (WHO 2002).

Prevention Generates Big Savings

Out of a desire to downplay the true cost, champions of universal coverage, have a tendency to overstate the financial returns from spending on prevention and wellness programs, as was apparent in the broad generalizations and overstated claims made by many presidential candidates in the 2008 national election (Cohen, Newmann, and Weinstein 2008: 661–63). Politicians believing that prevention is a pathway to large financial returns ostensibly are inspired by published reports pointing to such possibilities.

Several recent articles proclaim that nearly two-thirds of the rise in health spending over the previous two decades is traceable to such behavioral factors as overconsumption of food, lack of exercise, smoking, and stress. They allege that per capita health costs would be 30 percent lower if obesity levels had not increased over the past twenty years (Thorpe 2005; Engelberg Center for Health Reform 2009; see also US Senate, Health, Education, Labor and Pensions Committee Hearing, 2008). One group even claimed that health care spending could be cut by more than $16 billion within five years if as little as $10 per capita was invested annually on simple, tested wellness strategies such as affordable, nutritious foods, safe sidewalks and parks, and raising the tax on tobacco products. "Out of the $16 billion, Medicare could save more than $5 billion, Medicaid could save more than $1.9 billion, and private payers could save more than $9 billion" (Trust for America's Health 2008).

Reports like these find a receptive audience because the idea that prevention can save money has a commonsense appeal that makes people want to believe in them. The old adage that an ounce of prevention is worth a pound of cure is deeply embedded in popular culture. There indeed are savings to be had, but for the most part, they are transitory in nature. Over long periods, medical successes are transposed into higher costs. The paradox is that modern medicine makes it possible for people to survive who otherwise would have died, only to succumb later in life to more complicated and costly disorders. In the past people died when they got sick. Now they live sick. The prevalence of chronic disease and disability and the associated treatment costs testifies to the incongruity of medicine. Nowhere is this more apparent than at the neonatal level.

Survival rates for low birth weight infants have improved dramatically. The same applies to infants born with severe congenital disorders. In the past, such infants seldom survived beyond childhood. Today, for the most part, life expectancy has been extended to middle age. In both instance, however, the gains have been accompanied by a lifetime need for expensive social and health support services. The high cost of special education schooling is indicative. Annual per capita outlays for special education students are more than double that of ordinary students. Special education presently is said to account for roughly one-fifth of school budgets (Hechinger 2009: A4). Additional expenditures result from the cost of residential housing and related support services following the completion of schooling. These expenditures moreover do not include the cost of monthly disability payments that eligible disabled adults receive throughout their lifetime. To be sure, not all the disabled are unemployable. Examples of individuals who overcome serious handicap to become partially or fully self-supporting are an inspirational testimony to the power of perseverance and indomitable fortitude.

Among low birth weight survivors, many individuals require continuing medical attention and are susceptible to such conditions as hearing loss, blindness, cerebral palsy, and seizures. It is common for this group to be more susceptible to other health issues throughout life. For example, more than half of those with Down syndrome, over the age of 50, will develop early-onset Alzheimer's disease (Menendez 2005:

246–52). Approximately five million American children and adolescents have one or more conditions such as cerebral palsy, Down syndrome, spina bifida, congenital heart disease, pediatric brain tumors, stroke, epilepsy, autism, hearing impairment, or vision impairment that result in developmental disabilities. Impairments in cognition, speech, ability for self-care, and physical health persist throughout life hampering ability to carry out common daily tasks and necessitating supportive care. Lifetime costs from persons born in a single year with one or more of seventeen major birth defects are estimated at $6 billion. Some disabilities incur more cost because they require life-long care and special services.

The lifetime costs of infants born with mental retardation, cerebral palsy, hearing loss, and vision loss are estimated to amount to $260 billion measured in 2003 dollars (Boyle and Cordero 2005). Individuals on the autism spectrum are another example. They are believed to incur lifetime costs of $3.2 million. Caring for all persons with autism costs an estimated $35 billion per year (Harvard School of Public Health 2009). Fetal alcohol syndrome (FAS) is yet another costly birth defect. Lifetime medical and residential support services in excess of $2 million were projected in 2002 to care for children born with FAS, of which $1.6 million consists of medical treatment, special education, and residential care, and $0.4 million is due to productivity losses (Lupton 2003).

According to a recent Institute of Medicine study, preterm births also impose a heavy economic burden on society, one that amounts to at least $26 billion per year, or $51,600 per infant. About 12 percent of all pregnancies result in a premature birth that weighs less than 2,500 grams or 5.5 pounds (Institute of Medicine 2006). This problem is on the increase. Since 1980 the rate of preterm births has grown by more than 30 percent. While many social factors are involved, improvements in reproductive medicine are becoming a significant contributor. Recent advancements in fertility treatments have resulted in an increase in the number of multiple births that are at higher risk for a preterm delivery.

The actual cost attributable to premature births is much higher than reported above as it only includes the first five years of life following birth. When the treatment of all possible lifelong disabilities and years of lost productivity for the caregivers are factored into the costs, the actual expenditure may be more than $50 billion (Ante 2008: 47–49). Neonatal intensive care deservedly is widely hailed as a triumph of modern medicine. Medical advances now make it possible for babies weighing a little over one pound to survive who had no chance of surviving a few years ago. In most neonatal centers, survival rates approach 50 percent. Miraculous as this is, survival comes at a steep price. Daily hospital charges exceed $3,500 per infant, and it is not unusual for costs to total $1 million or more for a prolonged stay, much of which is borne by Medicaid given the correlation of low–birth rate pregnancies with low-income mothers. However, the cost goes far beyond initial hospitalization. Medicine has made little progress in reducing the high incidence of physical disability affecting surviving low–birth weight babies. Approximately one-fourth of all newborns younger than twenty-six weeks' gestation acquire a disability significant enough to affect their ability to function independently (Muraskas and Parsi 2008: 655–58). Modern medicine's paradoxical effect is not limited to the beginning stage of the life cycle.

At the other end of the life cycle, progress in medical diagnosis and treatment has transformed once important deadly diseases into chronic conditions. For example, diabetes formerly killed those afflicted with it—quickly in the case of children and slowly among persons diagnosed with it later in life. Today most people with diabetes look forward to a normal life span but require medication and medical monitoring. Treatment of cancer and heart disease has similarly improved. However, severe and costly cognitive and physical disabilities often are a side effect of successful treatment. Unless the right treatment is started within five to seven minutes following a heart attack, survivors experience brain damage. Cardiac surgery conveys a similar risk. More than half of the people who go through coronary artery bypass surgery suffer a significant postoperative decline in cognitive ability (Abramson 2005: 173). In the case of cancer survivors, heavy exposure to powerful radiation and chemotherapy can exact a heavy price in terms of quality of survival concerns. This also applies to those with AIDS. They experience major physical and emotional complications from side effects related to treatment options (e.g., see Gross 2008).

Among the terminally ill, the ability of medicine to prolong survival stirs debate and controversy for several reasons, one of those being the magnitude of spending involved. Spending on behalf of persons in their last year of life is five times greater than for those who are not in their last year of life. Among Medicare beneficiaries, roughly six times more is spent on persons in their final year of life than for other beneficiaries (Center for Medicare and Medicaid Services 2003). The magnitude of spending differentials is one reason why physician-assisted suicide, and the withdrawal of life support technology from the persons declared brain dead, are deeply entangled in disturbing right-to-life controversies besetting secular and religious communities.

As the percentage of the population entering the end stage of the life cycle continues to increase, pressures inevitably will mount for the federal government to assume greater financial responsibility for long-term care services that presently are paid mainly by the states and private households. Whereas acute care expenditures for physician and hospital services grow at a reduced rate as age of death increases, expenditures for long-term care do the opposite. Among the very old, age 85 and over, the probability of requiring costly nursing home and other forms of long-term care increase sharply, and as said earlier, the very old constitutes the fastest growing population group (Spillman and Lubitz 2000: 1409–15).

The limitations described do not apply to all preventive measures. The benefits of childhood immunization, of course, are a notable exception. The daily use of aspirin for the prevention of cardiovascular events for middle-aged patients is another. In both instances the cost of intervention is low and the long-term cost savings are large. On the whole, however, the alleged financial saving from prevention are inflated. The efficacy of many preventive services has not been clinically demonstrated and the economic implications are not well understood (Congressional Budget Office 2008). There are instances where a preventive intervention improves the length and quality of people's lives, but in the case of the elderly, it increases spending on Medicare and Social Security.

Preventive medicine, broadly defined, encompasses the benefits of early detection and management of chronic conditions as well as disease avoidance. For the most part, neither health screening nor disease management practices have been demonstrated to save money in the final analysis. Population disease screening saves money only in instances when the population susceptible to an illness is large enough to offset the cost of conducting the screening and treatment costs, along with other costs resulting from diagnostic errors. Errors in diagnosis may unnecessarily subject individuals to treatments that are not only costly but also unpleasant and even harmful. Most screening tests have low yields and even when the tests are highly reliable, the number of healthy people who are wrongly treated may exceed the number of persons who were correctly identified and treated (for a discussion of the shortcomings of medical screening, see Mechanic 2006).

Even highly accurate tests are problematic. Diagnostic technology in instances like CT screening for lung cancer, for example, is very accurate in detecting the smallest tumors. However, technology fails to recognize that the body's immune system prevents small ones from growing into large ones so that individuals identified with small tumors are subjected unnecessarily to risky surgery from which they may suffer serious complications (Bach et al. 2007). Much the same applies to screening for prostate cancer where the benefit of the prostate specific antigen test (PSA) remains unclear, and the cost and harmful side effects of overdiagnosis and overtreatment are substantial (Barry 2009).

A recently completed longitudinal study in Europe concluded that 1,410 men would need to be screened and an additional 48 would need to be treated in order to prevent one cancer death during a ten-year period (Schroder et al. 2009). Although there are many examples where prevention prolongs life and improves health, this is not the same as saving money. (For examples of how prevention does improve the lives of older people, see Russell 1987.) Yet another problem with screening is that it may misrepresent the benefits of early treatment. Improved five-year survival rates for breast and prostate cancers, for example, may have less to do with improved cancer treatment methods than to the identification of early-stage and often innocuous tumors. In other words, improvements in survival may be an illusion—neither cancer treatment or survival rates have actually improved (Welch, Schwartz, and Woloshin 2000; Baum 2000)

In summary, there is little reason to believe that preventive medicine in its present state is capable of generating the magnitude of savings in health care expenditures that often are suggested by proponents of universal coverage. As pointed out by Russell, over four decades of cost-effectiveness studies have conclusively shown that prevention usually adds to medical spending (Russell 2009). Yet proponents of government-financed health care continue to make exaggerated claims. There is a long history for this. Future health care savings were the chief selling point behind the enactment of England's National Health Service at the end of the Second World War. Spending, it was said, would level off and decline once the benefits of prevention took hold (Beveridge 1942). Over a half century later, this has yet to happen (*The Economist* 1998).

England's experience is a strong indication that the true value of prevention lies, not in the money to be saved, but in the reaffirmation of humanitarian values and the enhancement of quality of life. Sometimes the cheapest thing to do is to allow a person to die. The goal of health care is not to save money but to get the best value from what is spent. When cure is not possible, it signifies optimizing capacity for independent living by alleviating pain and discomfort, slowing the progression of disease, and compassionate end-of-life care. Blanket statements that prevention saves money are too simplistic. Sometimes it does, but as a rule it does not. Appeals to cost-saving potential are misguided. Instead of saving money, health care ought to be about allowing as many individuals as possible to lead fulfilling lives commensurate with their health status. (For a convenient and insightful reading on the limitations of prevention, see Verghese 2009: W1–W2.)

Universal Coverage Eliminates Social Disparities in Health Care

The contention that social disparities in health status and access to high-quality health care will disappear once universal coverage is implemented is overly optimistic. Real world obstacles seriously constrain, if not preclude, the attainment of egalitarian objectives. In light of the historic failure of highly motivated socialist and communist nations to eliminate social and economic disparities, any expectation that this can be accomplished in health care is unrealistic. More specifically, the failure of England's National Health Service in this regard is illuminating. Despite many concerted efforts England has been unable to do away with disparities in health status. Social and economic differences not only have persisted; they actually have widened in many instances, providing yet another example of the difference between theory and practice (Shaw et al. 2009; also Smith and Blane 1990; Department of Health and Social Security 1980).

Geographic and socioeconomic differences in the distribution and quality of health facilities and personnel are perpetuated as illustrated by the Inverse Need Law described above. Upper socioeconomic interests typically succeed in acquiring additional health resources. In this context, health does not differ from other desirable goods and services. Physicians and other health professionals are disproportionately attracted to high quality of life areas featuring cultural activities, quality schools for their children, and a safe environment. Therefore, while universal coverage may eliminate income and price barriers to health care, the services found in rural and low-income settings remain fewer and are of a lower standard than those available to groups that are more privileged.

This predicament, however, does not imply that it is useless to try to close disparity gaps so much as to underscore the difficulties involved. In persevering to address social disparities in health and health care, it is helpful to keep in mind the contribution of other factors. Ultimately the principal determinants of health lie outside the purview of traditional physician and hospital services. They include such things as bad dietary habits, personal hygiene, unsafe sex, tobacco use, alcohol and chemical dependencies, physical inactivity, and occupational and environmental hazards (Michaud et al. 2001). The significance of behavioral habits is accentuated by government-funded research indicating that half of all deaths occurring annually in the United States could be averted if people simply led healthier lives (Ding et al. 2009).

Clearly, the conventional view of the benefits of medical treatment is overly narrow and deterministic—a much broader view of the effects of living standards and behavioral factors is necessary. Continued belief that health is synonymous with health care is badly outdated. Income distribution and differences in education and other determinants of living standards contribute far more to health status than can be attributed to receipt of health services alone. They shape food consumption patterns, exposure to environmental hazards, and cultural differences in lifestyle behaviors (e.g., see Hertzman, Frank, and Evans 1994; Evans, Barer, and Marmor 1994). Upward social mobility serves to mitigate poverty's pernicious effects. However, mortality rates tend to be lowest in countries where income is more evenly divided, suggesting that relative deprivation may be even more important than absolute living standards (Wilkinson 1997).

In sum, public policy initiatives geared to economic growth and good paying jobs are essential components to any strategy for raising health levels and alleviating social disparities. However, it must be said that intergenerational poverty and the perpetuation of subcultures detrimental to educational attainment and social well-being do not readily yield to corrective measures. Progress typically is measured in decades and may require prolonged multigenerational commitments.

Health Services Are Safe and Efficacious

Contrary to popular perception, the health sector is lax when it comes to efficiency and quality control. The two are closely intertwined. Precise estimates remain elusive, but it is generally agreed that between 20 to 40 percent of all health spending is wasteful (Orszag 2008a; Cutler 2004).

Other reputable sources estimate the amount of waste as high as 50 percent (O'Neil 2007; PricewaterhouseCoopers 2008). In addition to the potentially large misallocation of money that could be better spent on improving access and other health reform priorities, wasteful spending also exposes individuals to considerable health risks.

More care is not always better care. In many instances more care is an indication of bad care. In regions of the country where chronic illness is treated more intensively than elsewhere, individuals are subjected to greater health risks, including the risk of dying. The factors believed responsible for this include receipt of care from multiple different physicians who seldom coordinate their care or clearly communicate instructions that are understandable to patients and their families, exposure to infections and medical errors from unnecessary hospital stays, and the incentive fee-for-service providers have to overprescribe and overtreat. This also applies to such serious conditions as heart attack and hip fracture (Wennberg 2008; Fisher et al. 2008).

The idealization of medicine as a profession in which patient welfare is paramount and the physician's hand is guided by a no-harm dictum belies the reality that health care treatment is a leading cause of death and disability. Most medical professionals when surveyed admit to having witnessed serious medical errors—95 percent of physicians, 89 percent of nurses, and 82 percent of health care executives (Wirthlin Worldwide 2001: 3).

Medication errors serious enough to cause injury occur 1.5 million times a year due to ineligible physician handwriting and faulty labeling and packaging along with other causes, including failure to check for medication side effects or the possible harmful interactions when multiple drugs are prescribed (Institute of Medicine 2006). The resulting annual deaths number around 7,000—about 16 percent more than the number resulting from work-related injuries. According to the Institute of Medicine (2000), somewhere between 44,000 to 98,000 persons are believed to die yearly from medical errors occurring in hospitals. However, this estimate may be far too low. The actual number of deaths is alleged to be far higher—around 200,000—than reported by the Institute of Medicine (2004). Even using the lowest estimate, medical errors rate as the eighth leading cause of death in the nation—higher than motor vehicle accidents, breast cancer, or AIDS (Agency for Healthcare Research and Quality 2009).

Due to a lack of systematic procedures for averting mistakes and a neglect of elementary germ control methods, hospitals have become dangerous to patients' health and, in many instances, no longer are the best sites for providing care. Government statistics indicate that the number of hospital-acquired infections is 1.7 million, or 4.5 hospital infections for every 100 patients. These infections are estimated to result, directly and indirectly, in nearly 99,000 deaths. Although most patients survive to be discharged, many endure years of treatment, multiple surgeries, and permanent disabilities (Klevens et al. 2002).

Surgical procedures are shifting to smaller ambulatory centers where infection rates are much lower for reasons including newness of facilities, avoidance of complicated medical conditions, and highly motivated, trained staff. This shift is made possible by innovations in minimally invasive surgical procedures (e.g., laproscopy, endoscopy, and arthroscopy) as well as financial incentives. Currently around two-thirds of all surgery is done in ambulatory surgical centers and another 13 percent is done in physicians' offices (McKinsey Global Institute 2008, 51).

Hospitals thus increasingly are being left with the more highly specialized complicated procedures. In many respects they are beginning to take on the appearance of massive intensive care units. The severity of the medical and surgical conditions they treat raises the risks of infection, since seriously ill patients often have compromised immune systems. This especially pertains to older patients who account for a growing number of hospital admissions. Patients risk acquiring life-threatening infections and serious harm from treatment errors that are due to nonexistent and faulty system controls and insufficient monitoring and oversight. Notwithstanding the gravity of the problem, little progress has occurred in reducing deaths attributable to medical errors in the decade following the Institute of Medicine's finding (Consumer Union 2009). This lack of progress underscores the difficulty of overcoming the many obstacles to change in health care, of which some of the more important are discussed below.

The traditional deference granted to the medical profession that is inherent in its status as a self-regulating and self-policing entity, along with the clinical autonomy physicians have long possessed in clinical decision-making results in insufficient accountability. These special properties commanded by the medical profession are fundamental to understanding the source of the problem but only provide a partial explanation. Self-regulation is intermixed with other factors. Foremost among these are the financial incentives physicians have to overprescribe. According to the Rand Corporation (2009), one-third or more of all medical treatment may be inappropriate. Contributing to this problem is the fact that physician income is determined by the volume and intensity of procedures performed instead of the appropriateness and results of treatment (Orszag 2008a).

Reimbursement incentives discourage hospitals and physicians from moving vigorously to address quality-of-care issues. It is indeed incongruous that health professionals are fully compensated for treating problems resulting from their mistakes. The re-hospitalization of Medicare patients is illustrative. Roughly one-fifth of hospital discharges in 2003 and 2004 were readmitted within 30 days and another 30 percent were re-hospitalized within 90 days. About 90 percent of these re-admissions were unplanned and involved high-risk issues such as heart failure, pneumonia, and gastrointestinal problems. These readmissions cost Medicare over $17 billion (Jenks, Williams, and Coleman 2009).

A better alignment of incentives and results would be an enormous help but once again falls short of solving quality-of-care concerns. Despite the perverse financial incentives, physicians often provide too little care, due to a lack of routinely applied good practice guidelines as well as a lack of financial rewards for adhering to them. Besides, inability to pay because of the nonaffordability of insurance coverage and other forms of financial hardship prevents many low-income people from seeking timely care. When eventually seen, they not only are sicker but, by the Inverse Need Law mentioned earlier, are treated in settings that are inferior to those serving persons who are not poor.

Beyond the influence of perverse financial incentives, the problem highlights the absence of uniform treatment standards to guide clinical decisions. Twenty to 30 percent of the care persons receive may be medically questionable or unnecessary. For many important medical conditions, patients fail to receive the proper treatment 50 percent or more of the time (McGlynn et al. 2003; Orszag 2008b). Adherence to good practice guidelines, while not a cure-all, would bring problems of over- and underutilization under better control by shrinking the scope of medically questionable and unsupportable variations in treatment practices. Related to the lack of uniform treatment protocols is the difficulty health professional encounter in acquiring convenient and reliable information on a patient's medical history that can be vital in selecting the right treatment.

Health care's image for scientifically driven advancement and technological prowess belies the rudimentary state of the data available to physicians. Among information intensive industries, health care is conspicuous for the slowness with which it is making use of the best information technology. Continued dependence on inconveniently stored and hard to read paper records promotes unnecessary duplicative tests and procedures, contributes to needless exposure to medication and surgical risks, and hampers safe and effective coordination of the inter- actions of the large number of staff involved in patient care.

Information technology exists that would make it possible for physi- cians to quickly access all the data required to help any given patient at any time and place. It also permits the integration of the many health components—physicians, hospitals, medical laboratories, pharmacies, and insurers—with potentially large gains in quality improvement. By linking all these components into a single electronic system, informa- tion technology enables researchers to search for correlations provid- ing vital clues as to treatment viability based on patient characteristics and the severity of medical conditions and complicating comorbidities. Equally important, the integration of clinical and financial information facilitates studies of cost-effectiveness, allowing researchers to deter- mine which treatments work best for the least cost (e.g., see *The Econo- mist* 2009).

Fear of loss of clinical autonomy and exposure to public scrutiny, although important, do not fully explain why the state of information technology lags so badly in health care. In fairness, the potential for cyber invasions of patient privacy and misuse of confidential medical histories to deny employment and health insurance coverage are valid concerns. Affordability is also an issue. The high cost of purchasing and maintaining information systems—ranging from $20 million to $100 million—strain the financial capabilities of all but the largest medical groups and hospitals (Agency for Healthcare Research and Quality 2006). Unlike other sectors of the economy where organizational size and concentration provides economies of scale, health care provid- ers are small sized, more numerous, and more dispersed. Costs vary widely, but for a midsized hospital they are estimated at $10 million over several years (Oldstein 2009).

It is no surprise therefore that health care remains in the entry stage of adopting modern information technology. It is estimated that as few as 17 percent of physicians and 8 to 10 percent of hospitals have any type of electronic medical record system and even fewer have and routinely use advanced models that allow for seamless exchange of information among key health care providers (Steinbrook 2009). Another survey found that only 1.5 percent of hospitals have electronic systems that are integrated in all clinical units of a given facility (Ashish et al. 2009).

Among hospitals without electronic record systems, purchasing and maintenance costs are the most commonly cited reasons, followed by physician resistance, uncertain return on investments, and lack of in-house information technology expertise (Ashish et al. 2009). There are unspecified but potentially large savings from more widespread use of health information technology by among other things, downsizing administrative and clerical staff, cutting the cost of delivering services, avoiding redundancies such as duplicative diagnostic tests, and improving providers' productivity. However, numerous practical barriers must be overcome before such savings can be actually attained. Many physician offices and hospitals remain too small to afford the acquisition and maintenance cost of integrated electronic systems. In many instances the efficiency savings come at the expense of provider revenues.

In fee-for-service reimbursement, for example, revenue is a function of the volume of care provided; therefore procedures that reduce the number of billings convey a financial disincentive against adopting them. This disincentive is a major reason why physicians and hospitals are slow to adopt health information technology (Rand Corporation Research 2009). The perverse effects of fee-for-service reimbursement also hamper improvements in the efficiency of laboratory and imaging services and quality-of-care improvements aimed at reducing unnecessary medical and surgical procedures.

At this stage of health sector development, the most auspicious settings for information technology are in large health care corporate entities that integrate outpatient and inpatient services and involve multiple hospitals and physician offices, such as Kaiser Permanente, Intermountain HealthCare, Geisenger Health System, and Henry Ford Health System. For large organizations like these, the annual cost of developing and running a modern information technology system is approximately 4 percent of operating costs, implying that it would require expenditures of around $50 billion per year to install and maintain health care information technology on a nationwide basis. Due to provider resistance and the costs involved, the Congressional Budget Office does not anticipate that more than two-fifths of physicians will adopt information technology by the year 2019 (Congressional Budget Office 2008).

Information technology is not only woefully underused in health care, but in instances where it is used, its usefulness is limited because differences in engineering design and software preclude standardized information from being conveyed between and among the full range of involved parties. The questionable quality of current generation software adds to the problems. Other than the Veterans Administration, applications of information technology to date have resulted in only marginal improvements in patient safety, largely because competition among suppliers leads them to push mass-produced software that requires time-consuming and expensive customization. Other problems stem from errors in data entry and confusing screens. In addition to debugging software, it will take time before all health personnel are comfortable with and competent in the use of information technology. Considering the potential, it is easy to overestimate the actual savings from information technology. Because solid evidence of the savings is not yet available, the Congressional Budget Office has made only modest projections (Congressional Budget Office 2008).

The British experience that is far ahead of US developments is indicative. An over $18 billion investment in digitalizing the entire National Health Service is running four years behind schedule because of software problems and vendor troubles. Reportedly, few British physicians are using electronic records and there is little evidence that they thus far have saved money or improved patient care. Supporters of digital medicine are predisposed to oversell the benefits of technology and to forget that more data does not always result in better health care (Terhune, Epstein, and Arnst 2009).

More and better information technology is essential, but it alone will not solve the health care quality problem. This is because ambiguity and uncertainty are a defining characteristic of health care and a reason why caution is advised in generalizing from comparisons with other economic sectors. Unpredictability in the way individuals respond to disease and treatment comprises the legitimate basis for the clinical autonomy status and wide latitude in treatment decisions granted physicians.

Except for the simplest medical conditions, unanimity of professional opinion on treatment of complex chronic conditions is rare, as exemplified in the multiple options for dealing with heart disease, prostate cancer, and breast cancer. Drug therapy presents a similar problem. Individual differences in response to treatment cause physicians to follow a trial and error process in drug selection and dosage. This partly explains why disease treatment costs vary widely both within and across geographic areas. An analysis of Medicare spending revealed that in some regions of the country it costs 60 percent more than in lower cost regions to care for patients with similar medical conditions (Fisher et al.

2003). When moving toward greater standardization of treatment protocols the advantages need to be balanced against the possible disadvantages. Allowance must be made for the fact that the natural course of disease and response to medical intervention differs among patients. A criticism of clinical guidelines is that they fail to allow for this and lead to cookbook medicine (e.g., see Cabana et al. 1999; Rutledge 2006).

Paradoxically, clinical autonomy is both essential to good patient care and a root cause of poor quality care as indicated in the following examples: Physicians commonly order legal prescriptions for uses other than those previously approved by government regulation. This practice adds to the risk of harmful side effects inherent in all medications. Despite concerns about patient safety and the added costs, there is a paucity of information about the frequency of off-label prescribing, including the amount of supporting scientific evidence. A study of the prescribing of 160 common drugs found that off-label use accounted for about one-fifth of all prescriptions, and in nearly three-fourths of the time the off-label use was shown to have little or no scientific evidence (Radley, Finkelstein, and Stafford 2006; Stafford 2008). Off-label use varies considerably by medical specialty. It is believed to total 30 percent of psychiatric prescriptions and as much as 75 percent of prescriptions written by pediatricians (Walton et al. 2008). Estimates of off-label prescribing possibly runs as high as 60 percent of all written prescriptions (Mehlman 2005).

Another disquieting aspect of clinical autonomy is that it allows an unknown but large number of physicians to perform complex medical procedures for which they are unqualified, or that they perform too infrequently to maintain recommended skill levels (Dudley 2000; Birkmeyer 2002; Birkmeyer et al. 2003; Kizer 2003; Peterson et al. 2004). Hospitals are expected to control quality through the granting and supervision of medical staff privileges, but enforcement is inconsistent due to management failures, some of which emanate from the hospital's dependence on income generated by medical staff who are independent practitioners and not hospital employees, assigning too low a priority to quality control, or ineffective management. Historically hospital administrators have acquiesced to medical authority and not taken a strong leadership stand on this issue preferring instead to concentrate on facilities management and financial affairs.

It is only recently that graduate training programs in health care management have elevated the importance of this responsibility to professional management (Battistella et al. 2005). One can anticipate that hospital management will become more assertive as the number of physicians working full-time in hospitals increases. Although only about 10 percent of physicians are now employed by hospitals, it is expected that 25 percent will become hospital employees by 2013 (Kennedy, Scoll, and Collier 2009).

Currently the financial pressures hospitals are under place heavy demands on the time of senior management and drive them to concentrate on manipulating the reimbursement system. Medicare payments, for example, are higher and more profitable for surgical procedures such as heart bypass than for pneumonia and other medical admissions. Differences in the profitability of individual services direct staff recruitment and the incorporation of technologies that are geared more to profit margins than to quality improvement and the community's medical needs (Ginsberg and Grossman 2005).

The subjugation of quality control to malpractice litigation is yet another obstacle to the establishment of quality improvement procedures. Malpractice litigation feeds a psychology of anxiety and intimidation that invites concealment of medical errors. Whether or not seldom invoked, the cost of litigation and the severity of possible sanctions, such as public humiliation and loss of licensure, precludes using errors as a learning instrument. Within this culture of blame, physicians and other health providers fear leaving an incriminating paper trail to be exploited by contingency fee lawyers. Consequently a considerable percentage of medical errors is never disclosed (Roscoe and Krizek 2002).

Wald and Shojania (2001) indicate that only 1.5 percent of all errors results in an incident report, and only 6 percent of adverse drug events is identified properly. The American College of Surgeons, as reported by Wald and Kaveh (2001) states that only 5 to 30 percent of surgical errors are reported and only 20 percent of surgical complications is included in weekly quality review sessions. Clearly, continued reliance on malpractice litigation as a means of holding physicians accountable for the quality of care they provide is reactionary. The time has arrived to replace this coercive practice with positive incentives that are conducive to an environment of ongoing learning and improvement.

In the final analysis, balancing legitimate physician concerns for clinical autonomy with the need for long delayed improvements in performance accountability and transparency is unlikely to succeed if physicians are seen as the cause of the problem rather than as partners in devising solutions. Without their full cooperation and participation, progress in efficiency and quality improvement will be compromised

(Battistella and Weil 1998). As discussed earlier, the authority physicians command over diagnosis and treatment contains the power to make or break managerial objectives for reducing cost and upgrading patient care standards.

Beyond physician cooperation, the reliability and accuracy of information for the development of medical standards and clinical guidelines is indispensable to creating an infrastructure supportive of effective quality control methods. Underscoring this is the finding that less than half of all medical treatments is substantiated by scientific evidence as being effective (Institute of Medicine 2007). Also reported is that although heart disease is among the most studied illnesses in all medicine, half of the medical treatment recommendations is based largely on medical opinion and has not been subjected to vigorous scientific testing (Pierluigi et al. 2009).

Better evidence on what works best under different patient care circumstances and on cost-effectiveness of treatments is central to obtaining major reductions in the number of unnecessary procedures and substantial savings while at the same time improving patient care. Ultimately evidence-based medical treatments are only as good as the data from which they are derived. It is a challenge to obtain accurate and reliable clinical data, however. The importance of doing so is underscored in the recent initiative to establish a national program for supporting better decision-making about interventions in health care. The American Recovery and Reinvestment Act of 2009 allotted $1.1 billion in support of comparative effectiveness research (Iglehart 2009b).

Because of difficulties inherent in conducting clinical research, much of the evidence supporting evidence-based therapies is less reliable than commonly supposed. Ethical restrictions on the use of human subjects in medical research that limit randomized double-blind clinical trials are a case in point. Thus the value of surgical interventions necessarily relies mainly on observation and opinion.

The most exacting research practices are usually confined to drug studies. Even in the most prestigious medical journals, much of what is published is suspect. Deficiencies of research design, insufficient sample size, and exaggeration of the practical as distinct from statistically significant findings undermine the utility of the information. A particularly notorious example of this is the widespread public alarm and costly lawsuits triggered by the erroneous finding first published in *The Lancet* that autism is linked to the childhood measles, mumps, and rubella vaccine (Begley 2009).

All of this is compounded by potential conflict of interest issues in the surprisingly large number of instances where researchers fail to disclose ties to commercial firms standing to benefit from positive study findings (e.g., see Abramson 2005: 93–100; Angel 2000; Armstrong 2008; Korn 2000; Weintraub and Barrett 2006; Winstein 2009). The seriousness of this problem is underscored by the recent commissioning of the Institute of Medicine to study and report on how to prevent bias and mistrust. In addition to urging greater disclosure of individual and institutional financial ties to industry, the report called on medical institutions to standardize procedures for assessing the severity of conflicts and how to deal with them in order to restore confidence in self-regulation. Self-regulation was upheld as an alternative to government intervention that might stifle an otherwise socially beneficial relationship between industry and medical professionals (Lo and Field 2009). The problem goes beyond these types of conflicts of interest.

Pressures on those conducting research interfere with the application of rigorous scientific methodologies. Clinical investigators whose careers depend on publishing and obtaining grants are subject to ethical lapses involving data falsification, and the withholding and underreporting of negative findings (Chen 2008; Chen et al. 2004). Often data are examined to find interesting effects, and after-the-fact hypotheses are constructed rather than formulating them in advance. Similar ethical lapses apply to research organizations having a vested financial interest in the outcome of research findings. Because of limitations such as these, it is estimated that up to 50 percent of all scientific papers are flawed (Ionnidis 2005).

Studies adhering to the gold standard of randomized clinical trials are no less free of limitations. The cost and complexity of enlisting and retaining human subjects limits the number and frequency with which they can be conducted. An even bigger problem stems from the length of time required to complete clinical trials. Periods of a decade or more are not uncommon, and by the time the study is published, the medical treatment under investigation has changed to an extent that the findings no longer are relevant. According to the Tufts Center for the Study of Drug Development, the cost of bringing a new drug to market totals over a billion dollars currently and the process takes from five to ten years (Tufts 2009; Knowledge@Emory 2003). Excluding overhead expensed, it cost pharmaceutical firms around $6,000 for each person it enrolls in a clinical trial (Emanuel et al. 2003). Clinical trials involve several phases, and each phase can involve thousands of patients. The phase 4 study of Viox, for example, included over 8,000 people (Abramson 2005: 33–36).

Summary

Single-payer universal coverage will not attain the savings proclaimed by its proponents. When assessed in light of real world constraints, single-payer coverage falls considerably short of being fiscally responsible. It is founded on expressions of faith that are disconnected from evidence. The large expansion of spending required is not recoupable from investments in preventive services and in health status, and there are innumerable difficulties in micromanaging anything as complex as health care through centralized planning and control. The complexities are compounded by the uncertainties inherent in medical research and clinical practice that limit the extent to which policy can be guided by scientific research findings.

These considerations are a reminder that many of the assumptions and beliefs that have dominated health policy deliberations are outdated and need to be reassessed in the light of the new demographic and economic realities that are straining both government and employer financed health care to the point of collapse. Dealing with today's health care issues necessitates a paradigm shift whereby the primacy of ideologically driven policy-making defers to practical considerations of cost-effectiveness and affordability.

6 Health Policy Reconfigured

The escalation of public debt, coupled with the size of unfunded entitlement obligations, signals a need for government restraint and financial responsibility in the undertaking of expensive new programs. Financial constraints on employment-based coverage are perilous to ignore under existing circumstances. Employers can no longer be the main source of protection against the threat of household financial insecurity that results from the high cost of health care. In today's economic environment employers have far less flexibility to offset higher benefit costs by such traditional practices as raising prices or lowering wages. If still possible in the long term, competitive pressures for economic survival limit finding interim solutions in sufficient time to avoid competitive disadvantage and loss of business and a steady erosion of employer-provided health insurance.

Collectively bargained contract obligations, for example, limit what can be done in the immediate future. One need only consider the plight of American automobile manufacturers and the problems resulting in the restructuring of the US steel industry attributable to labor wage and benefit agreements for active workers and to retiree health benefits (Lowenstein 2008). In light of the constraints on government and employer spending, practicality foretells the need for greater exploration of formerly repudiated shared responsibility whereby individuals are expected to participate commensurate with their ability to pay. How employers, government, and consumers can be expected to participate in the unfolding of health reform is the subject of this chapter. The chapter concludes with an appeal for a new health policy paradigm.

Based on the nature of health care issues and trends analyzed in preceding chapters a number of conclusions appear evident:

• Employers will cease being the primary source of health insurance coverage.

• The federal government lacks the capacity to take on sole responsibility for financing new and costly entitlement programs.

• The idealized version of national health insurance, including its single-payer counterpart, is an idea whose time has passed.

• The equalitarian principles undergirding Medicare that prohibits differential treatment by income are fast eroding. Upper income beneficiaries will be required to contribute more and receive less. Full benefits will be paid only to those who truly need them; all others will be cut back.

• Cost containment strategies that fail to share efficiency savings with consumers are unlikely to succeed.

• Constraints on government and employer financing indicate that entirely free health care is unrealistic.

• The post–World War II period, whereby household out-of-pocket health care spending steadily declined, is unlikely to continue. If anything, households will be required to share responsibility for financing health care based on ability to pay.

• Government will recognize its inability to micromanage health care and focus instead on setting standards and overseeing programs.

The failure of earlier domestic efforts to modernize health care, in combination with the problems other high-income nations are encountering in financing and managing their health care systems, strongly suggests the need for a new health policy paradigm in which lofty aspirations are tempered by a greater appreciation for practical limitations.

Different Employer Health Care Role

Business and industry are in the process of redefining their traditional role in the provision of health coverage. No longer will they serve as a first line of defense in protecting individuals and families against the cost of health care. Government subsidies that established employers in the past as the principal source of health insurance coverage are insufficient to offset the disadvantages employers encounter in performing this function. As mentioned earlier, the financial plight of domestically owned automobile manufacturers is a clear indication of the burden of providing employee health coverage under conditions of an aging labor force and large retiree population. Because of the correlation between age and the incidence of illness and disability, firms having a young workforce pay less for experience-rated health insurance premiums than counterparts whose workers are older. This is becoming a generic problem as the entire population is in the process of aging.

Most Americans still receive health insurance through their employers. Ninety percent of persons have private health insurance coverage through employer-provided plans. Whether it remains in the national interest to press for a continuation of this arrangement is doubtful. The cost of providing this benefit hinders competitiveness and profitability, leading employers to economize either by reducing their role in financing employee coverage or by discontinuing the benefit. Health insurance is the largest nonwage component of total compensation amounting to one-third of expenditures on voluntary employee benefits and 7 percent of total payroll (Federal Reserve Bank of San Francisco 2009).

Increasingly employers who remain committed to continuing health insurance coverage for their workforce are shifting more of the cost to employees through means of premium charges, deductibles, and coinsurance requirements, while scaling back or eliminating retiree health coverage. Among the changes, retirement health benefits are the most severely affected. Between 1993 and 2001 employer coverage for early retirees declined from 46 percent to 29 percent, and coverage for Medicare eligible retirees declined from 40 percent to 23 percent (Employee Benefit Research Institute 2002; Kaiser Family Foundation 2004; McCormack et al. 2002).

Many employers are pursuing more innovative means for providing affordable health care. They are concentrating employee coverage on major medical expenses, transforming health insurance from a defined benefit to a defined contribution plan patterned after precedents established in the provision of employee pensions, and enlisting employees as stakeholders in cost containment (Watson Wyatt 2009). For small-sized firms searching for affordable ways to continue providing employee coverage, health savings accounts are becoming an attractive option (Fronstin 2008).

Cost containment strategies vary according to employer size. High premium costs deter small firms from offering health insurance, since premiums correlate inversely to group size. Not only do small-sized groups pay higher premiums, they evince greater premium instability. Premiums assigned by insurers can jump up astronomically following one or more incidents of workers incurring large hospital and physician charges when treated for serious illness or a maternity case involving costly intensive neonatal care. It is common in such instances for a firm with fewer than twenty-five employees to have its premium increased by 50 percent or more and have its insurer withdraw coverage at contract renewal time, thus forcing the firm to search for a new insurer.

Many small employers who provide coverage may cut back on the level of protection or disengage entirely, thereby adding to the size of the nation's uninsured and underinsured problem. Employees may choose to reject the shifted costs of coverage once out-of-pocket requirements cut too deeply into take-home pay. Cost shifting to employees particularly affects low-income workers who unfortunately are most in need of protection against potentially high health care costs.

The speed at which the employer as the main source of insurance declines coverage is relative to the state of the general economy. That is to say, when workers and their dependents most require the security of health insurance coverage, it becomes less reliable and a source of worker anxiety: when jobs disappear, insurance coverage disappears with them. This lack of security is a serious limitation that results from reliance on employer-provided health insurance. An increase in the number of uninsured is only one of the undesirable economic repercussions that flow from periods of economic decline and volatility.

Loss of employment and insurance coverage leads both to a rise in the volume of uncompensated care borne by hospitals and other health providers and to pressures to expand Medicaid enrollments. Unfortunately, large increases in uncompensated care usually happen just when state governments are under pressure to cut expenditures—when they can least afford to expand Medicaid enrollments. Hospital annual uncompensated care runs close to 6 percent of expenses. In 2007 the national total amounted to $34 billion. Normally public hospitals are disproportionately impacted, but during severe economic downturns the burden on hospitals is more broadly shared (American Hospital Association 2008).

Reliance on employers to provide insurance has the additional disadvantage of hindering job mobility to the detriment of the nation making better use of labor resources. Unevenness in the availability and comprehensiveness of coverage provided by firms discourages individuals from switching jobs for fear of being without coverage while searching for a new job, or working elsewhere where benefits are lower or nonexistent. Such fears naturally multiply during periods of economic turmoil when good paying jobs are scarce, causing individuals to forgo opportunities where they could be more productive.

Federal law allows a continuation of employer coverage for a period of eighteen months upon leaving or losing a job. Over 70 percent of persons having this option chose to reject it principally because they have to pay the entire premium plus a two percent administrative fee when they can least afford it (Fronstin 1998). Moreover, when persons exercising the eighteen-month coverage option seek and are approved for individual coverage, they generally are priced out of that market. Although insurers are legally prohibited from basing premiums on preexisting conditions, they nevertheless have wide latitude in setting rates. In 2008 the average family premium for an eligible unemployed worker amounted to 83 percent of unemployment income (McCanne 2009).

Apart from the high cost, this temporary benefit is not available for persons laid off from very small companies since employers having fewer than twenty employees are exempted. Other exclusions apply to workers in firms that never offered health insurance, have terminated plans or have gone out of business. To ease the pain of recession-related unemployment, the American Recovery and Investment Act of 2009 (ARRA) provides a 65 percent subsidy for up to nine months for eligible individuals (http://www.irs.gov/newsroom/article/0,,id=204505,00 .html). To qualify, a worker has to have been involuntarily separated between September 1, 2008, and December 31, 2009.

Individuals wishing to continue insurance coverage following the expiration of the eighteen-month period encounter yet higher premium costs if they do not succeed in obtaining a job that provides health insurance. Once no longer covered by their former employer's group plan, they have recourse only to more expensive individual coverage. Group policies are far less expensive because the number of healthy persons enrolled offsets or neutralizes outlays required to pay for the care of unhealthy enrollees, and actuarial predictability increases with group size. Additionally group enrollment permits economies in marketing and administrative costs. Group enrollment in fact protects insurers against adverse risk selection.

On the assumption that individuals who seek coverage on their own do not do so unless they either have a present health need or anticipate having one in the near future, insurers charge more in order to cushion against higher underwriting risks. It also explains the practice of excluding coverage for preexisting medical conditions. In comparison, uninsured healthy persons are inclined to roll the dice. The risk of not finding or being unable to afford available coverage makes it harder for individuals to take on the challenge of starting a new business or taking on a new job that may be a better fit. It also discourages individuals from early retirement. Insofar as labor immobility impedes small business start-ups and productivity improvement, it is socially dysfunctional.

In the modern economy, lifetime job tenure is fast becoming a condition of the past. Not only is frequent change of employment becoming the new norm; more individuals may become self-employed in the future. Also temporary and part-time employment is growing as firms seek greater flexibility in staffing and savings in fringe benefit costs, all the more so during periods of economic downturn (Lee and Mather 2008). The self-employed do not easily fit into the traditional pattern of employment-based coverage, and they have trouble finding affordable health insurance. Together with individuals who work as freelancers, consultants, or independent contractors, they already comprise close to one-third of the nation's workforce. The best way for them to obtain affordable coverage is by forming or joining a group specifically designed for obtaining lower cost health insurance, an option that is only now becoming more available (e.g., see Freelancers Union 2009).

Ironically, the large financial incentive the government gives employers to encourage them to make coverage available to their employees is part of the problem. The cost to the US treasury of excluding insurance premiums from taxable income was around $200 billion in 2007, a sum that was more than half of what the federal government spent on the Medicare program. However, this money is not well spent (Kaiser Family Foundation 2008). Because of the way the tax code is structured, this results in high-income families obtaining broader and better coverage than low-income families and leaves the self-employed in a position where they have too little, if any, assistance. High-income individuals are employed disproportionately in firms that are more profitable and therefore offer benefits that are more generous. Since employers are not taxed on the money they spend on health insurance, it is an inducement for them to provide employees with more coverage than they otherwise would. Thus high-income individuals acquire gold-plated policies, while employees in less profitable firms get less generous benefits, if any at all.

While it is true that all employees receiving health insurance benefit because, unlike wages, health insurance is not taxed as a form of income, high-income employees benefit more. Given that the tax value of the benefit is directly related to income, they get a bigger tax break than do low-income employees. Therefore, when an employer spends $10,000 on a policy, it provides employees in the highest income tax bracket with about a $4,000 exclusion (Gruber 2009).

Employment-based health coverage thus discriminates against low-income individuals and the self-employed. It also deters the long-term uninsured from purchasing private health coverage following the loss of employment due to corporate layoffs and downsizing, since they do not get an equivalent tax subsidy. This particularly pertains to individuals who are unlikely to get another job because of their age but are too young to qualify for Medicare (Lyke 2008).

Given the disadvantages of the present method of providing the labor force with insurance coverage, a restructuring of existing tax incentives is inevitable. To align employment-based health insurance with the reality of today's job market, health insurance must not penalize the unemployed and entrepreneurial-minded workers who are motivated to start their own business. In brief, this requires a transfer of ownership of health insurance from employers to employees so that job mobility is facilitated rather than stifled. Accomplishing this objective necessitates a major revamping of health insurance tax subsidies so that the benefits go directly to individuals rather than indirectly through employers. The value of tax benefits also has to be fairly structured to assure that all income groups are treated equally (Fronstin and Salisbury 2007).

Short of outright transfer of ownership, the tax benefit may be redirected to reduce income inequalities in the availability and scope of coverage while also lowering the cost of health care. If a ceiling were imposed on the tax benefit, workers expectedly would press employers to offer health plans valued at or below the limit. Employees would only have to pay taxes on the value of coverage that exceeded the cap. Employers then would offer less comprehensive plans that, in addition to lowering coverage inequalities, would help curb excess demand for health care (Fronstin 2009). According to Feldstein, the free-good effect of current tax rules raises private health spending by as much as 35 percent (Feldstein 2009). Moreover, as providing health insurance becomes less burdensome, there will be less pressure on employers to shift health cost to employees or to discontinue coverage.

End of Open-Ended Government Health Spending

Government does not have an unbounded capacity to absorb additional entitlement health spending. Because of the present size of unfunded future obligations for Social Security, Medicare, and Medicaid, government already has promised more than can be delivered without drastically revising eligibility and benefit provisions. Within less than a decade the Medicare program will start paying out more in benefits than it receives from payroll taxes (O'Sullivan 2008). To compensate for this shortfall, Congress will have to make painful choices apropos of curtailing spending for other programs, increasing the national debt through borrowing, or raising taxes. Arcane government accounting rules will cause this to begin decades prior to the date it officially runs out of money.

If left in their present form, Medicare, Medicaid, and Social Security will consume a disproportionate share of the federal budget and drastically squeeze the amount of revenues available for other government programs. Together, these three programs already comprise over two-fifths of federal outlays (Penner and Koch 2007). Interest payments on the national debt run close to 9 percent. Another fifth is committed to defense spending that, because of international tensions and threats to national security, is unlikely to be scaled back any time soon. Together with smaller programs like veterans' benefits, mandatory spending accounts for over 70 percent of the federal budget. This leaves approximately 25 percent to fund all remaining government functions. This amount will decline further due to faster growth in the big three entitlement programs (Social Security, Medicare, and Medicaid) as the baby boomer generation retires.

The health spending problem is exacerbated by the fact that, due largely to medical innovation, it is growing faster than the economy. Once the baby boomer wave passes in 2030, the population will go on aging as life expectancy continues to grow and birth rates remain low by historical standards (Kotlikoff and Burns 2004: 1–39). The cost of financing the federal deficit will grow sharply beyond its present level due to the extraordinary amount of borrowing by the federal government to jump-start the economy during recessionary periods. Thus the amount of the budget remaining for other government functions is destined to become even smaller in future years (Budget of the US Government 2009).

Expanding health care entitlements as envisioned in single-payer health care or national health insurance adds to the nation's long-term financial dilemma—all the more so when the unfunded future liability for Social Security, Medicare, and Medicaid is added to the mix. Although commonly reported as $40 trillion, this unfunded future obligation of the federal government is actually closer to $50 trillion when the estimated cost of the new Medicare drug benefit is included. Yet another $2.3 trillion unfunded liability exists for medical and disability benefits promised to civil servants and military personnel. From a technical standpoint, such an amount is enough to bankrupt the nation as it exceeds the nation's net worth. The size of this outstanding bill is the neighborhood of $600,000 per household, an amount that if not paid off currently will become larger when paid with interest over time (Kotlikoff and Burns 2004: 244; also see Cauchon 2006). As a share of GDP the amount of national wealth going to Social Security, Medicare and Medicaid will rise from 8.4 percent in 2008 to 18.6 percent by 2050. In comparison, the entire 2008 federal budget is 20 percent of GDP (Orszag 2008).

From the standpoint of federal revenues required to meet the deficits from Social Security and Medicare, the problem seems even more formidable. Unless the government rescinds or modifies its promises, the deficit from these two programs will equal 25 percent of federal income taxes in fifteen years. The government will have to either raise taxes by an equivalent amount or borrow the money to fund the programs. The problem will only worsen. By 2030 the midpoint of the baby boomer retirement years, the combined deficits will equal roughly 40 percent of federal income taxes (Greenspan 2007: 414). The cost of paying this obligation is staggering. As reported by Kotlikoff and Burns (2004: 54), paying for these two programs alone will require doubling the payroll tax by 2030, and tripling it sometime near 2075.

Clearly, raising payroll taxes to fund universal coverage, a major expansion of entitlement obligations, is not a financially responsible option. Payroll taxes are highly regressive. They already impose a heavy burden on low-income and middle-income workers. Roughly half of taxpayers pay nothing or very little in individual income taxes (Sorensen and Cobb 2000). Payroll taxes are a major reason why workers' wages have stagnated in recent years and in many cases failed to keep up with inflation. Most economists agree that virtually all of the payroll tax ultimately comes out of the pockets of workers, including the portion paid by employers. When looked at in this way, the combined 15.3 percent payroll tax for Social Security and Medicare surpasses what workers in low tax brackets pay in income tax.

Among households in the bottom 20 percent of the income scale, the average payroll burden in 2006 was $917 while the average income tax payment amounted to $171. For middle-income households, payroll taxes are nearly double on average what they pay in federal income tax. Among the bottom 40 percent of households, income taxes are less significant than payroll taxes, property taxes or state or local sales taxes

(Prante 2007). The prospect of resorting to income taxes to pay for the Social Security and Medicare deficit is more enticing but destined to end in disappointment. Increasing taxes by 10.2 percent of GDP now would amount to $1 trillion or $12,072 per household and require raising income tax rates by 120 percent or more. For households in the 35 percent tax bracket, taxes would have to go up close to 80 percent and for those in the 25 percent tax bracket, by at least 55 percent (Riedl 2008).

Taxing the rich to pay seems a straightforward and fair way to raise the necessary funds. However, this is a deceivingly simple solution. Just who qualifies as rich is less easily quantifiable than popularly assumed. After immediately dismissing the bottom half of taxpayers whose incomes are generally considered too low, the question of whom to target remains highly subjective. Families making less than $50,000 certainly do not see themselves as rich. The same applies to families in the $100,000 category. Families living in major metropolitan areas find that housing, infant care, saving for children's college tuition, and other expenses, including state and local taxes, stretch household income after paying federal income taxes. Many in higher income brackets feel the same, thereby possibly shrinking the pool of targeted taxpayers down to the top 10 percent or smaller. Independent of any successful political opposition from income groups finally selected, there is absolutely no way (Kotlikoff and Burns 2004: 54) their taxes can be raised high enough to collect all the money needed. In the end everyone will have to pay.

Taxing employers more is equally unfeasible. Having them contribute more in payroll taxes only compounds the disadvantage firms already encounter when competing against foreign rivals in lower labor cost countries. Raising corporate income taxes also detracts from profitability and competitiveness. It fosters perverse incentives for firms to invest in and retain profits outside the United States. In recent years governments in most other industrial countries have been lowering corporate taxes to a point where they now are below the current US rate. Raising corporate and personal taxes to levels that will ameliorate, if not solve, the entitlement funding crisis runs the risk of discouraging work, savings, and investment and encouraging capital flow abroad or inciting all manner of tax avoidance and evasion behavior.

Since income and payroll taxes in their current form cannot be relied on to provide the necessary funds, policy makers will have little choice but to drastically reform the tax code. Some methods of doing this include eliminating the plethora of popular tax deductions such as home mortgage interest payments, instituting a flat tax, or turning to sales taxes, in which case accommodations will be required to deal with the regressive impact on low-income households.

Avoiding the problem will only makes matters worse. A delay of fifteen years, for example, adds another $25 to $30 trillion to the amount outstanding, due to the cumulative effect of interest payments. Regrettably, there is no painless fix to this problem. Neither economic growth, nor immigration, nor eliminating waste, fraud, and abuse provide much help. Nor is it realistic to expect that it will be possible to continue borrowing from the Chinese, Japanese, and other foreign creditors. Except for lenders from the Middle East, their populations are aging faster than in the United States, so they will have to direct more of their savings internally (Organization for Economic Cooperation and Development 2005). In addition to changes in the price of oil, the availability of credit from oil-exporting Middle Eastern countries will decline as they begin to diversify their economies and make the necessary investments to create good jobs for their disproportionately young populations.

Unless something is done, tomorrow's generation of US taxpayers will have to pay taxes that are two or more times higher than current rates. In addition to entitlement program liabilities, there is the large national debt that must be dealt with (Kotlikoff and Burns 2004). Resolving the unfunded entitlement programs requires bold measures. While helpful, any recalibration of Social Security's cost of living allowance formula that slows increases in annual payments will be insufficient. As Kotlikoff and Burns (2004) see it, a partial privatization of Social Security is unavoidable. With respect to Medicare and Medicaid, the economy measures increasingly cited involve eliminating fee-for-service provider reimbursement and limiting payment to new medical technologies that meet cost-effectiveness testing. (Daschle 2008: 155–57; Benson 2008; Walker 2004).

Some politicians and economists argue that the seriousness of the entitlement financing issue is overblown and that only minor changes are required—any problems can be largely solved by stimulating faster economic growth through a combination of tax cuts, productivity improvements, and borrowing. For this to happen, according to the Government Accountability Office, requires that GDP grow at a double digit rate for the next seventy-five years—a highly unlikely eventuality considering that economic growth averaged less than 4 percent during the 1990s (Walker 2008).

Because of the enormous difficulty, the federal government faces in balancing its budget for the near future, converting Medicare and other publicly funded programs to some type of voucher system will become a politically attractive means of imposing greater budgetary discipline. Vouchers simplify reform by circumventing dependence on bulky bureaucratic mechanisms intrinsic to alternative reform proposals. Above all else, they enable government to plan for health expenditures in advance of the fiscal year while allowing recipients a measure of freedom of choice in their selection of an insurer. The advantage of bureaucratic simplicity combined with a minimum of interference with individual freedom of choice suggests that the federal role in financing universal coverage will proceed in this direction.

Briefly stated, voucher payments would be sufficient to provide a basic set of essential health benefits patterned after the previously described FEHBP plan for government employees and members of Congress. Participating insurers would be required to accept everyone regardless of preexisting health conditions and guarantee renewal each year (Emanuel 2008). In order to compensate for differences in need for financial assistance because of differences in health status, the value of vouchers could be adjusted so that healthy individuals receive a smaller voucher payment than persons having a costly medical condition (Kotlikoff and Burns 2004: 143–71).

Change in the way entitlement programs are funded also appears inevitable. The entitlement financial problem is a consequence of its reliance on the pay-as-you-go principle. As previously described, every dollar collected is spent without any investments being made to pay off future obligations. Promises are made on the assumption that succeeding generations are willing and able to pay higher taxes than today's workers pay.

This assumption, however, becomes more tenuous as future taxes attain punitive levels and young persons of working age begin to question, as currently is happening, whether they will receive the same benefits when they retire or indeed whether the programs will still be in existence (e.g., see Friedlander 2005; Belt 1999; Rasmussen 2009). Moving to a funded system, where worker contributions are saved and invested, averts this issue. This is why some thirty countries have already begun or completed the process of changing their pay-as-you-go-systems into partially or fully funded systems (Goodman 2005).

National Health Insurance Outdated

The conventional model of national health insurance, or single-payer coverage as it has been relabeled, is no longer viable. It has been overtaken by the realities of an aging society and the financial consequences of the nation's long-term habit of saving too little, spending too much, and being overdependent on foreign creditors. Overdependence on foreign credit seriously constricts the government's ability to manage the economy insofar as it reduces latitude for adjusting fiscal and monetary policy to changing macroeconomic conditions. If, in paying off the debt, the government prints money to help inflate the problem away, creditors may insist on higher returns to protect the value of securities they hold, thereby thwarting government efforts to reduce debt-service charges.

Due to the size of unfunded future entitlement payments, and the impracticality of large tax increases and borrowing, it is imprudent for government to take on the financing of a major increase in entitlement spending until the economy returns to normal (Greenspan 2007: 409–22). The government's inability to contain Medicare spending serves as a warning. It is a single-payer plan whose costs have become unsustainable.

If stymied by political obstacles single-payer enthusiasts may revert instead to a stealth strategy for achieving their goal. The idea is to gradually reach a tipping point where a sufficient percentage of the population is covered by public plans so that efficiency and equity issues compel creating a single government plan for the entire population (e.g., see Sparer 2009). Growth in the size of the uninsured population due to recession related unemployment feeds such aspirations (e.g., see Angeles 2009). However, this strategy of creeping universalism, no matter how clever, is equally unrealistic. While the political equation may become altered in the process, the financial constraints remain unchanged.

Notwithstanding federal cost sharing, the states, as described earlier, are in an even weaker position than the federal government when it comes to being able to assume major increases in health care spending. States are already struggling to meet their present Child Health Insurance and Medicaid obligations. In order to cope, many states now require that Medicaid beneficiaries pay something when they receive medical care. These out-of-pocket payments have become substantial and are growing twice as fast as increases in beneficiary income and faster than those for persons with private health insurance. The only beneficiaries spared these charges are children and pregnant women (Broddus and Ku 2005).

Nor, as discussed above, is it realistic to expect that employers can be made to pay more for health care. The competitive challenge characterizing the new economy prevents them from expanding beyond present levels of involvement. Even adhering to the status quo poses a challenge. Economic realities being what they are, the employer role in health care is more apt to decline than expand. This will be accelerated should mandatory private health insurance coverage proposals levy financial penalties on employers for discontinuing employee coverage that are significantly less than what they pay in insurance premiums, thereby providing them with an incentive to get out of the business of providing health insurance.

Disintegration of Medicare's Equalitarian Foundation

Financial pressures are chipping away at the equalitarian-egalitarian foundation of entitlement programs. Medicare is in the early stages of withdrawing from its historic commitment to a single standard of rights and benefits for all without distinction to differences in social and economic status. The scaling of Part B physicians and outpatient premiums to income foretells a movement toward selectivity in eligibility and benefit standards. One can anticipate that the Part D prescription drug component will follow a similar path. Yet other dissimilarities point to greater selectivity in the Medicare program

Low-income elderly burdened by out-of-pocket Medicare charges receive special assistance. In both Parts B and D they qualify for enrollment in a dual eligibility program whereby such costs are borne by Medicaid. For low-income persons whose incomes are too high to automatically qualify for Medicaid, government subsidies help defray the cost of premium and other out-of-pocket charges in the drug benefit program (Department of Health and Human Services 2009). Another socioeconomic distinction centers on the range of choices available beyond the basic fee-for-service option that confers advantages to better-educated and better-informed Medicare beneficiaries. Greater differentiation of benefits will be hard to avoid as budgetary restrictions reconfigure Medicare into a multi-tier health care system.

The plight of low-income elderly is especially ironic. Protecting the elderly against health care costs seen as a main cause of income insecurity and poverty provided the moral impetus for Medicare legislation, but this liberal impulse has since succumbed to fiscal exigency. In order to postpone the date of trust find insolvency, Medicare has enacted numerous increases in Part B premiums and cost-sharing requirements that have reintroduced income insecurity and poverty within low-income elderly households. These payment requirements have pushed close to two million elderly with incomes or resources just above the federal poverty line to seek Medicaid relief where they became part of the seven million seniors already on the Medicaid rolls.

Roughly 15 percent of the elderly were enrolled in Medicaid in 2005. Together with non-elderly disabled persons who also qualify for Medicare coverage, they accounted for nearly one-fifth of Medicaid enrollment and 46 percent of Medicaid expenditures for medical services. Of this amount, 20 percent went toward Medicare premiums and cost sharing. Long-term care and other services not covered by Medicare accounted for most of the reminder. Thus cost shifting to the elderly also compounds problems the states have in budgeting for Medicaid. Had the federal government fully funded Medicare premiums in 2005, it would have reduced state Medicaid spending by nearly $4 billion (Holahan, Miller, and Rousseau 2009).

More of the near-poor elderly for whom Social Security is their primary source of income will fall into poverty in future years if Medicare premium increases continue to outpace Social Security cost-of-living allowances as they have been doing since first instituted. For decades premium increases have been depleting elderly discretionary income because of this discrepancy. Unfortunately, other than an occasional year when Medicare premium increases are withheld, there is no indication that the situation will improve. Between 2001 and 2006 Medicare premiums increased at an average of 12 percent a year (Social Security Law Attorney 2006). In comparison, Social Security payment increases averaged less than 3 percent a year (Social Security Online Fact Sheet 2009).

The bottom line is that Social Security will replace a smaller percentage of the average worker's pre-retirement income. The amount will gradually fall from a present level of 39 percent to about 32 percent over the next several decades (Greenstein 2009). While a problem for the elderly the gap will become an even greater problem for the young if premiums continue to rise at their historic rate.

Medicare cost-saving measures may precipitate yet more problems for the elderly. Dismayed by cuts in reimbursement approved, but not yet acted on, by Congress, many physicians are thinking of ending their relationship with Medicare or limiting the number of Medicare patients in their practice. This threat has not materialized to date because the government keeps postponing the scheduled cuts in physician reimbursement. Nevertheless, the frustration of having to cope with government regulations and reimbursement rates below those received from private insurers has led some to refocus their practice on high-end fee-for-service clients.

Although involving few physicians thus far, the emergence of boutique or concierge medicine nevertheless spawns worries of a continuing deterioration of Medicare coverage if and when planned cuts in reimbursement are enacted (US Government Accountability Office 2005). An attraction for physicians is that in this type of practice they can see half as many or fewer patients without experiencing any loss of income. In reducing provider reimbursement, the government risks having health providers sever their ties to Medicare. This would significantly compound the problems the elderly have in obtaining medical care.

The magnitude of foreseeable budgetary and financial strains limiting the growth and stability of public programs is a reason for taking a more critical look at the right-to-health-care doctrine in terms of setting boundaries consistent with the limitations on government spending. The already frayed policy of extending government-funded free care to persons able to pay privately is likely to continue unraveling. The precedent of paying full benefits only to persons who really need them and cutting back on payments to everyone else is already well established. Along with enabling government to focus limited resources on the poor, requiring the wealthy to pay for more of their own coverage puts individuals who are best equipped in terms of education and sophistication in the forefront of attempts to have health providers practice greater cost restraint.

Targeting social benefits in this manner is not something unique to the United States. Faced with equally if not more severe financial constraints, the British National Health Service, as mentioned earlier, has been steadily moving away from the ideal of universal, comprehensive health care that is equally available to all and disconnected from income and ability to pay. That this shift has acquired the endorsement of a left of center government underscores the gravity of the entitlement funding issue (Pollock 2004). Yet other countries long envied by reformers for their progressive welfare state policies have embarked on similar changes. Both Finland and Sweden are targeting benefits along these lines in order to maintain the solvency of retirement and health programs (Cowen 2008). While Canada remains committed to single-payer health care, the system is encountering severe financial strain, raising concerns about its sustainability. In Ontario, close to half of the government's spending goes to health care, an amount that is expected to continue to increase in future years. This is precipitating a search for financing alternatives (Flood, Stabile, and Tuohy 2008: 1–36).

While certainly not a welfare program, the federal–provincial partnership at the core of the Canadian system ironically otherwise closely parallels the federal–state US Medicaid partnership in matters of administration and financing, with the result that both are encountering comparable issues of uniformity of benefits and financial sustainability. Not only has the junior partner financial burden grown to the point of crowding out other public services as the result of health inflation and political pressures to expand benefits beyond the minimum required, but in both instances the loss of revenues during times of economic recession compounds the financial strains that threaten to dissolve the arrangement.

Although the frequent subject of partisan criticism and challenge, efforts to privatize Medicare, particularly through financial incentives for increasing the role of managed care organizations, will not dissipate. Rather, privatization is more apt to take on new forms, such as the Federal Employee Health Benefit Plan (FEHBP) model in which the elderly are granted vouchers to spend on pre-screened and pre-approved health plans (e.g., see Emanuel 2008). Rather than decreasing, the roughly one-third of Medicare recipients now enrolled in managed care plans may actually increase because self-interest provides an inducement for low- and moderate-income elderly to seek high-value plans containing fewer out-of-pocket payment requirements and better benefit coverage than contained in conventional Medicare fee-for-service coverage.

Consumer Partnership Vital to Cost Containment

Successful cost containment requires collaborating with consumers by allowing them to share in efficiency savings. The failure of cost containment to date is grounded in the inflationary dynamic inherent in third-party reimbursement. It disconnects individuals from the economic consequences of their utilization choices while at the same time inducing profligate billing practices among providers who are guaranteed payment. Because of the psychological illusion that health care is a free good, consumers not only tolerate excessive provider charges but behave with a comparable lack of self-restraint in the demands they place on health providers. This free-good mindset is reinforced by philosophical and moral convictions that are entrenched in the culture of health care and in the politics of national health insurance. In other words, the incentives are backward. Both consumers and providers are rewarded for overusing health care and reap none of the financial benefits from saving money.

Financial discipline will remain an elusive health care goal until the financial incentives are realigned to reward savings. Harnessing the power of self-interest and severing the consumer-provider spending alliance is an important first step. A transfer of health insurance ownership from employers and government to individuals and permitting them to share in any efficiency savings is vital for imparting price consciousness and prudent health services use. As consumers move from an enabler to a watchdog role, they will serve as a check on questionable provider pricing and billing practices.

High deductible health plans and tax advantaged health savings accounts, though still in their infancy, are an important step in this direction. Vouchers can be made to serve a similar purpose by devising payments so that given a choice, individuals have an incentive to select insurance plans on the basis of efficiency and quality. The unfolding of performance-based compensation methods and the halting of reimbursing physicians and hospitals for medical errors are recent developments that auger a more enlightened reform trend.

Household Responsibility

Necessity signals that households' role in paying for health care will not decline. If society has an ethical obligation to ensure universal access to quality health care, individuals, as recognized by a national commission concerned with health reform back in the mid-1980s, have a commensurate responsibility to pay for a fair share of the cost of their own health care commensurate with their ability to pay. The responsibility of the federal government is to ensure that those who otherwise cannot obtain adequate care are able to do so, and that the costs of care are shared equitably (President's Commission 1983).

In light of the magnitude of current financial constraints encountered by government and business and industry, individuals not securing coverage from employer or government programs will be mandated to do so privately. The fact that, as described earlier, a significant number of uninsured persons can afford to buy health insurance on their own supports this development. If enacted, proposed public subsidies and tax incentives to assist low-income households purchase health insurance would make such a requirement affordable to all while relieving insurers from the risks of adverse selection that otherwise causes them to reject sick persons or charge them more (Meckler and Fuhrmans 2009: A4). In this connection, policy makers increasingly are drawn to some

variation of the Massachusetts mandatory purchase model (Massachusetts Trial Court Libraries 2009).

The Massachusetts plan essentially eliminates the "free-rider" problem inasmuch as it compels everyone to have health insurance. It requires everyone, except the poor, to pay something. In order to make
coverage affordable, premiums for low-income persons are subsidized
on a sliding scale basis based on their income level. Individuals obtain
insurance either from their employer or private plans. Employers who
fail to offer coverage are assessed annual financial penalties. Financial
penalties are also applied against individuals who chose to remain uninsured. When first proposed in the early 1990s as a way to deal with
the uninsured problem mandatory household responsibility seemed
too heretical to be taken seriously. It speaks to the growth of awareness over the limits to federal financing that it now enjoys considerable
bipartisan support. For an early description of this approach, see Battistella and Kuder (May–June 1993 and Summer 1993).

Criticism that subsidies often are insufficient to avert financial stress
among middle-income households and that it is unfair to penalize them
for failing to purchase coverage they cannot afford is a valid concern.
Limiting total approved household health expenditures to a percentage
of disposable income would be a fairer method, but possibly infeasible
because of the accompanying administrative complexities. Nevertheless, continuing consolidation of the insurance industry into fewer
large-sized companies may soon render this issue irrelevant. Consolidation spurred by mandatory purchase will increase the risk-absorption
capacity of insurers as larger enrollments enable greater actuarial predictability and economies of scale result in lower and more affordable
premiums.

Over 400 health insurance mergers occurred between 1998 and 2008
to the effect that only two insurance companies presently cover one-third
of the entire insured population. In thirty-eight states, the largest firm
now controls one-third or more of the market; and in sixteen states the
largest firm controls more than half the market. In every state but California and Nevada, the largest insurer is a Blue Cross or Blue Shield
plan or both. Together the Blues plans and the three largest non-Blues
carriers have more than a 60 percent market share in thirty-four states
and more than 70 percent market share in twenty-three states (Arvantes
2007; Picker 2008; Robinson 2004).

While concentration normally is something to be eschewed as socially
harmful, the regulatory provisions contained in proposals requiring

individuals to purchase adequate coverage—for example, guaranteed issuance and premium pricing restrictions—offset the risks and converts bigness into a social benefit. By including all the young and healthy, mandatory purchase also insulates insurers from adverse-selection risks and puts an end to such socially dysfunctional practices as selective enrollment, discriminatory health status pricing, exclusion of preexisting conditions and post-enrollment waiting periods prior to the onset of full coverage. To the extent that sick and older enrollees are unevenly distributed, disadvantaged insurers can be properly compensated through means of special government payments.

Insurers moreover have an interest in devising more affordable individual health policies containing better health cost protection. As the result of large employers self-insuring and small-sized firms discontinuing health insurance benefits, the group policy market that has been the mainstay of the insurance industry is declining. Other than fees collected from managing corporate health benefit programs, the individual policy market is the only remaining growth area (McQueen 2008; Center for Market Intelligence 2009). Albeit selling of individual policies is more complicated and expensive than group policies, insurers are quickly learning how to deal with the challenge. Along with drawing on their experience with Medicare Advantage plans, they are absorbing lessons from the financial services industry, which had to make a comparable transition when employers began shifting from defined benefit to defined contribution plans.

Additionally health insurance industry consolidation, coupled with changes in the ownership of health insurance policies, will stimulate a greater sense of urgency for the development of uniform national standards to replace presently uneven and archaic state government regulation of health insurance firms, and expedite legislation favorable to the establishment of consumer-friendly health insurance purchasing groups. The establishment of uniform standards within the confines of a national market would vastly expand the scope and effectiveness of competition. It would accomplish more at less cost and complication than installing a public plan in each state to compete with private insurers. A net effect of these changes is that health insurers will become more like public utilities.

Government Intervention

Demographic and economic realities disincline government from expanding direct financial responsibility for health care. Consequently the financing of Medicare and other government health programs will become secondary to the formulation and advancement of policy objectives through standard setting and oversight activities. The federal government has little choice. As the large baby boomer generation enters the retirement stage, entitlement spending will consume money otherwise available for remaining government programs and services. This together with the cost of servicing a large national debt incurred during years of excessive borrowing will accelerate pressures to rein in entitlement spending. Financial constraints portend an end to retrospective open-ended Medicare and Medicaid financing.

Politically unpopular budgetary controls, along with public dislike of economy measures restricting freedom of choice and the rationing of access to costly high-technology medical procedures, makes elected officials uncomfortable for they estrange relations with constituents and endanger re-election prospects. Conditions therefore tilt in the direction of conceding and actively supporting a large private-sector role in which household responsibility is more apt to grow than diminish. Again, given the new realities, mandatory individual purchase of insurance coverage looms as the only practical avenue for the attainment of universal coverage. Privatization of universal coverage does not eliminate the need for government financing. In outsourcing responsibility to the private sector, the cost to government will nevertheless be substantial.

Estimates of the annual cost of subsidizing the insurance premiums for low-income persons runs as high as $100 billion to $150 billion in new federal spending per year or more (The Commonwealth Fund 2007; Sheils and Haught 2003). Being in a secondary role, however, is far less costly than assuming the entire cost of financing universal coverage. The assumption of a secondary role moreover enables elected officials to concentrate government capabilities on setting standards, monitoring private-sector performance, and evaluating efficiency and quality improvement practices.

Revised Health Policy Paradigm

An outdated attachment to a populist vision of unlimited free health care within an economy of boundless affluence underlies the aspirations of the single-payer health care movement. This disconnect from the true state of the economy and the enormity of the government's financial problems points to the need for a policy paradigm better attuned to today's realities. There is little to be gained from trying to solve today's health reform issues with yesterday's beliefs about how health care ought to be financed and delivered.

As said earlier, it is unrealistic to expect that government alone is the solution to the uninsured problem. Nor is it realistic to believe that the government is best equipped to manage the health sector. Politicization and paralysis of decision-making is difficult to avoid in a partisan political arena, and it is extremely optimistic to assume that politicians are in a position, given all the other demands on their time, to adequately comprehend the innumerable complexities peculiar to the management of health services. The vast number of ill-defined Medicare regulations is illustrative. They are the cause of countless differences of interpretation that sow confusion, induce errors, and provide a fertile environment for evasion and fraud.

Shifting health insurance ownership from third parties to individuals, a formerly heretical proposition is an idea that now seems less radical. In addition to removing an important barrier to labor mobility and better allocation of human capital, individual ownership imparts a heightened sense of cost consciousness and more thoughtful reflection on whether and where to seek health care. When considered in the light of the failure of past efforts to contain costs, health care savings accounts and related concepts such as vouchers merit dispassionate assessment. Notwithstanding often strident opposition, enlisting consumers as partners in cost containment by financially rewarding them for making prudent use of health services is slowly but steadily acquiring legitimacy.

Disapproval of market competition in health care also needs to be rethought. Its incremental spread over the past several decades commonly is incorrectly interpreted as a form of right wing ideological subversion (Richmond and Fein 2005: 129–57; Relman 2007). What is lost in this view are the repeated failures of government-directed regulatory and planning initiatives to modernize what was universally agreed to be a badly antiquated health care infrastructure. By taking decision-making out of politics and circumventing lengthy and costly due process delays, while also providing incentives that reward initiative and innovation, market competition has expedited and accelerated industry consolidation and the integration of modern managerial and corporate practices.

Market-oriented policies have also propelled employers to take a more active part in using their purchasing power and managerial expertise to facilitate the diffusion of modern efficiency and quality improvement methods. Large corporations, motivated to slow increases in employee health coverage expenditures, are largely responsible for improvements occurring in a number of important quality improvement areas. These include disease management, evidence-based medical standards, computerized prescription ordering, electronic records, medical report cards, provider profiling, system-based models (e.g., six sigma and other statistical methods derived from manufacturing controls) for medical error reduction, and hospital emergency room and intensive care staffing with physician specialists.

Greater awareness of the constraints of government financing is pushing policy makers to think more creatively about how the power of private interest can complement and assist government in the attainment of public policy objectives like universal coverage. As seen in health reform proposals recently sponsored by influential Democratic members of Congress, private financing is now viewed as a desirable adjunct to overstretched public resources. Their embrace of mandatory health insurance purchase with fines for noncompliant households is an even bigger break from the Party's historic attachment to orthodox national health insurance principles (see proposals introduced by Baucus and Wyden 2008; Wyden 2007). This break with Party orthodoxy was especially obvious in the 2008 presidential primary when all of the leading candidates for the Democratic nomination rejected the single-payer panacea (Iglehart 2009a).

Conventional beliefs and assumptions concerning how physicians and patients relate also need to be rethought. The characterization of the patient as a victim of uncontrollable circumstances, as someone who is intellectually incapable of comprehending clinical information and who furthermore is too overcome with emotion to act rationally in choosing among treatment options, is an out-dated conceptualization of the doctor–patient relationship. This is especially noticeable in norms instructing the surrender of consumer sovereignty to medical authority. This view belies the vast changes in intergenerational educational levels and cultural attitudes for personal autonomy and assertiveness that have narrowed once formidable knowledge gaps. Individuals are now encouraged and assisted in assuming greater responsibility for their health care decisions.

The ease with which information is acquired in today's information age facilitates the ongoing transformation of the individual from a patient into a consumer (Herzlinger 2007). Parallel changes that have lowered barriers to the role of market forces in health care complement and reinforce this transformation, as does the transition in disease patterns from acute-communicable to chronic-degenerative disorders. The array of choices for the treatment of chronic illness not only underscore the reality of medicine as an imperfect science that was obscured in the past when the population was less well-informed but constitute an invitation for individuals to assume greater responsibility in clinical decisions. Increased individual participation is generally endorsed and encouraged by the contemporary medical community—it reduces the incidence of malpractice litigation but, more important, increases patient's compliance with medical instructions.

Financial instruments like health savings accounts and vouchers prod individuals to pay more attention to health maintenance and empower them to challenge questionable provider pricing and billing practices. The power of self-interest inexorably leads health care consumers to place a premium on value and ultimately requires providers to compete on price and quality.

This motivational environment is conducive to a revival of not-for-profit managed care plans. Those providing comprehensive integrated care tend to outperform for-profit rivals on measures of value (Tu and Reschovsky 2002; Himmelstein et al. 1999; Kuttner 1998). Given a choice among competing health plans, financially astute consumers are more likely to accept restrictions on freedom of choice if the decision is theirs to make rather than imposed on them by others. (Regarding a possible revival of managed, see, for example, *The Economist* 2009: May 30, 12–14.)

If, as feared by opponents of multi-tiered health care, managed care growth becomes a predominantly low-income phenomenon, it nevertheless would represent a significant advancement of the pre-paid ideal extolled by reformers since the mid-1930s (Gray 2006). Granted a larger opportunity to demonstrate its superiority, managed care could appeal to upper income groups as well, in which event market competition, which is anathema to health reformers, ironically will have succeeded where altruistic exhortations and moral persuasion have failed.

Sanctioning an important role for the private sector in health care, while helpful, is not a cure for the wide range of outstanding equity and efficiency issues confounding health care. Rather, the significance lies in acknowledging, on the one hand, the futility of pursuing ideals and the practical value and, on the other hand, of harnessing the power of self-interest in endeavors for the common good. Surely this is the lesson to be derived from the repeated failures of single-minded, ideologically driven quests for national health insurance.

Pragmatism, in company with a multipronged strategy for cost containment and quality improvement, offers a promising avenue for achieving universal coverage. Closer attention to issues of affordability and the barriers to efficiency and quality improvement is a necessary precondition for resolving the uninsured problem. Balancing competing priorities for equity and economy presents an unending dilemma. Calculations of the trade-off between the desirable and the attainable require a policy climate favorable to trial and error and the flexibility to supplant what fails with what works.

Condemnation of market competition belies its widespread presence and perpetuates the political polarization that has stalemated past health reform initiatives. It also hampers understanding of the decision-making complexities that await students preparing for careers in health services policy and management. Their ability to function effectively upon attaining leadership status rests on an ability to accept and cope with the competing and contradictory service ethic and commercial signals routinely encountered in health care. The scope of private-sector involvement in health care is large and unlikely to disappear in the foreseeable future.

Notwithstanding the enormous difficulties involved, health policy and management needs to accommodate rather than denounce the confusion from the juxtaposition of contrasting incentives and rewards. Enlightened policy, at the end of the day, centers on an open-minded and tireless pursuit of creative synergies and the formulation of a paradigm that is attuned to the social and economic forces reshaping health care.

It is instructive to note that the movement toward a pragmatic acceptance of what was formerly dismissed as radical or iconoclastic is not isolated to the United States. It is common to many nations who are urgently seeking to control health costs while improving access to quality health care. Today there is wide support for health reforms that share responsibility among public and private payers. Only a minority of leaders in Canada and Europe continue to believe that tax revenues alone can sustain a health care system. New realities stemming from the high cost of new medical treatments, population aging, and the globalization of trade and commerce underlie a trend toward convergence in health policy featuring the creative use of market incentives for the application of modern managerial methods in health services structure and delivery (PricewaterhouseCoopers 2005).

In conclusion, health policy has reached a turning point. The influence of ideology that has dominated past disputes over health reform is fading. Increasingly policy makers are defying popular orthodoxies and accommodating new realities. New realities compel a re-examination of underlying conventional assumptions and beliefs on how best to finance and deliver health care. For similar reasons, liberal and conservative disputes that have deterred efforts to introduce modern managerial principles to correct antiquated efficiency and quality control practices are steadily being relegated to the margins in favor of more practical approaches.

Frustration over the stalemate in health reform attributable to the polarizing effects of ideologically driven solutions pushes decision makers to subordinate the ideal in favor of the practical. The visible trend toward a higher regard for pragmatism and practicality reflects the emergence of a more intellectually sober understanding of the inflationary ramifications of implementing idealized versions of universal free health care.

References

Aaron, Henry J. 1996. Health care reform: The clash of goals, facts, and ideology. In *Individual and Social Responsibility*, ed. Victor R. Fuchs. Chicago: University of Chicago Press, 107–35.

Aaron, Henry J. 2003. The cost of health care administration in the United States and Canada: Questionable answers to a questionable question. *New England Journal of Medicine* 349 (8): 801–803.

Aaron, Henry J., and William B. Schwartz. 1984. *The Painful Prescription: Rationing Hospital Care*. Washington, DC: Brookings Institution.

Abramson, John. 2005. *Overdosed America: The Broken Promise of American Medicine*. New York: Harper Perennial.

Adamy, Janet, and Elizabeth Williamson. 2009. As Congress goes on break, health lobbying heats up. *Wall Street Journal*, August 5: A1, A9

Agency for Healthcare Research and Quality. 2006. *Costs and Benefits of Health Information Technology*. US Department of Health and Human Services. Evidence Report/Technology Assessment 132. Publication 06–E006. April.

AMA (American Medical Association). 2009. Anti-euthanasia, pro-pain control. http://www.pregnantpause.org/euth/amagomez.html.

American Health Insurance Plans. 2007. 4.5 Million enrolled in health savings account plans, April 2. http://www.ahip.org/content/pressrelease.aspx?docid=19314.

American Health Insurance Plans. 2009. Center for Policy Research. February. http://www.ahipresearch.org/pdfs/PreliminaryAnalysisHSAsv2.pdf.

American Hospital Association. 2008. Uncompensated Hospital Care Cost Fact Sheet. November.

American Society of Plastic Surgeons. 2008. Quick facts. http://www.plasticsurgery.org/Media/stats/2008-quick-facts-cosmetic-surgery-minimally-invasive-statistics.pdf.

American Society of Plastic Surgeons. 2009. My plastic surgeon USA. Industry leaders, analysts forecast cosmetic plastic surgery market surgeons. http://www.myplasticsurgeonusa.com/articles.php?art=176.

Anderson, Gerard F., and Bianca K. Frogner. 2008. Health spending in OECD countries: Obtaining value per dollar. *Health Affairs* 27 (6): 1718–27.

Anderson, Odin W. 1958. Proposals for National Health Insurance: 1910–1950. In *Medical Care*, ed. Committee on Medical Care Teaching. Chapel Hill: University of North Carolina Press, 621–28.

Angell, Marcia. 2000. Is academic medicine for sale? *New England Journal of Medicine* 342 (20): 1516–18.

Angell, Marcia. 2009. Are we in a health care crisis? PBS interview. http://www.pbs.org/healthcarecrisis/Experts_intrv/m_angell.html.

Annas, George J. 1998. A national Bill of Patients' Rights. *New England Journal of Medicine* 338 (10): 695–99.

Appleby, Julie. 2000. Studies look at issue of immigrants, insurance. Center for Immigration Studies. *USA Today*, July 18. cis.org/articles/2000/coverage/newscoverage.html.

Arrow, Kenneth J. 1963. Uncertainty and the welfare economics of medical care. *American Economic Review* 53 (5): 941–73.

Arvantes, James. 2007. Insurer consolidation hurts health care quality, blocks access. American Academy of Family Physicians. http://www.aafp.org/online/en/home/publications/news/news-now/government-medicine/20071029kingtestimony.html (accessed October 29, 2007).

Auerbach, Alan, and William Gale. 2009. The economic crisis and the fiscal crisis: 2009 and beyond. Paper presented at the Brookings Institution, Washington, DC, March 8.

Austin, Andrew D. 2008. Trends in discretionary spending. CRS Report for Congress. Congressional Research Service, March 26.

Bach, Peter B. 2009. Limits on Medicare's ability to control rising spending on cancer drugs. *New England Journal of Medicine* 360 (6): 626–33.

Bane, Mary Jo, and David T. Elwood. 1994. *Welfare Realities*. Cambridge: Harvard University Press.

Battistella, Roger M. 1972. Rationalization of health services: Political and social assumptions. *International Journal of Health Services* 2 (3): 331–48.

Battistella, Roger M. 1986. Politics of government supported health services: Necessity for a new approach. In *Restructuring Health Policy: An International Challenge*, ed. John M. Virgo. Edwardsville, IL: International Health Economics and Management Institute, 55–70.

Battistella, Roger M. 1997. *The Political Economy of Health Services: A Review and Assessment of Major Ideological Influences and the Impact of New Economic Realities in Health Politics and Policy*, 3rd ed., eds. Theodor Litman and Leonard S. Robins. Albany, NY: Delmar, 75–108.

Battistella, Roger M., and David Burchfield. 2000. The future of employment-based health insurance. *Journal of Healthcare Management* 45 (1): 46–56.

Battistella, Roger M., and David Burchfield. 2003. Consumer-directed health care: Three options, one reality. *Employee Benefit Plan Review* 57 (12): 13–16.

Battistella, Roger M., and John M. Kuder. 1993. Universal access to health care: A practical perspective. *Journal of Health and Human Resources Administration* 16 (1): 6–34.

Battistella, Roger M., and Thomas P. Weil. 1998. Linking physician and nonphysician management roles in the managed care era. In *Search of Physician Leadership*, eds. Barbara LeTourneaua and Wesley Curry. Chicago: Health Administration Press.

Baum, Michael. 2000. Survival and reduction in mortality from breast cancer. *British Medical Journal* 320 (7274): 895–98.

Begley, Sharon. 2009. Anatomy of a scare. *Newsweek*, March 2.

Belt, Bradley D., ed. 1999. *The 21st century retirement security plan. National Commission on Retirement Policy Final Report*. Washington, DC: Center for Strategic and International Studies.

Benko, Laura B. 2003. Pitching plans to the uninsured. *Modern Healthcare*, February 24: 8–9.

Berge, Wendel. 1958. Social organization of medical care. In *Readings in Medical Care*, ed. Committee on Medical Care Teaching. Chapel Hill: University of North Carolina Press, 666–76.

Berman, Eric S., and Elizabeth K. Keating. 2006. *The Elephant in the Room: Unfunded Public Employee Health Care Benefits and GASB 45*. Boston: Pioneer Institute for Public Policy Research.

Bittle, Scott, and Jean Johnson. 2008. *Where Does The Money Go? Guide Tour to the Federal Budget Crisis*. New York: Harper Collins.

Blendon, Robert J., and Mollyann Brodie. 1997. Public opinion and health policy. In *Health Politics and Health Policy*. 3rd ed., eds. Theodor J. Litman and, Leonard S. Robins. Albany, NY: Delmar, 201–19 .

Blumenthal, David. 2009. Stimulating the adoption of health information technology. *New England Journal of Medicine* 360 (15): 1477–79.

BMC Health Services Research. 2006. Extent and structure of health insurance expenditures for complementary and alternative medicine expenditures, October 11. http://www.pubmedcentral.nih.gov/articlerender.fcgi?artid=1617102.

Boulding, Kenneth E. 1981. The concept of need for health services. In *Economics and Health Care*, ed. John B. McKinlay. Cambridge: MIT Press, 31–50.

Brenner, M. Harvey. 1987. Relation of economic change to Swedish health and social well-being, 1950–1980. *Social Science and Medicine* 25 (2): 183–95.

Brenner, M. Harvey. 1997. Heart disease mortality and economic changes: Including unemployment; in Western Germany, 1951–1989. *Acta Physiologica Scandinavica*, suppl. 640 (5): 149–52.

Broddus, Matt, and Leigton Ku. 2005. Out-of-pocket medical expenses for Medicaid beneficiaries are substantial and growing. Center on Budget and Policy Priorities, Washington, DC. May 31.

Brookings Institution. 2008. Taking back our fiscal future. Members of the Brookings-Heritage Fiscal Seminar. Brookings Institution, Washington, DC. April.

Cabana, Michael D., Cynthia S. Rand, and Neil R. Powe. 1999. Why don't physicians follow clinical practice guidelines? *Journal of the American Medical Association* 282 (15): 1458–65.

Cannon, Michael F., and Michael D. Tanner. 2005. *Healthy Competition*. Washington, DC: Cato Institute.

Cantor, Julie D. 2009. Conscientious objection gone awry: Restoring selfless professionalism in medicine. Perspective. *New England Journal of Medicine* 360 (15): 1484–85.

Carney, Brian M. 2009. The Weekend Interview with Judd Gregg. *Wall Street Journal*, April 25: A9.

Catalano, Ralph. 2009. Health, medical care, and economic crisis. *New England Journal of Medicine* 360 (8): 749–51.

Cauchon, Dennis. 2006. Huge bill for public retirees hits soon. *USA Today*, May 18. http://www.military-quotes.com/forum/promised-government-entitlements-will-cost-t21594.

Center for Market Intelligence. Health care plans northern light. http://www.ama-assn.org/amednews/2009/01/26/bisa0126.html.

Center for Responsive Politics. December 2008. http://www.opensecrets.org/lobby/top.php?showYear=2009&indexType=c.

Center on Budget and Policy Priorities. 2006. A brief overview of the major flaws with health savings accounts, April 5. http://www.cbpp.org/cms/index.cfm?fa=view&fa=222.

Chopra, Deepak, Dean Ornish, and Andrew Weil. 2009. Alternative medicine is mainstream. *Wall Street Journal*, January 9: A13.

Churchill, Edward D. 1958. The Hospital As A Social Institution. In *Readings In Medical Care*, ed. Committee on Medical Care Teaching. Chapel Hill: University of North Carolina Press, 256–67.

Cohn, Jonathan. 2007a. *Sick*. New York: Harper Collins.

Cohn, Jonathan. 2007b. What's the one thing big business and the Left have in common? *New York Times Magazine*, April 1: 45–49.

Committee for Economic Development Research and Policy Committee. 2002. *A New Vision for Health Care*. New York: Committee for Economic Development.

Coalition, Concord. 2009. U.S. national debt clock, March 13. http://www.brillig.com/debt_clock/.

Congressional Budget Office. 2008a. *Budget Options*, vol. 1. Washington, DC: Health Care.

Congressional Budget Office. 2008b. Key issues in analyzing health insurance proposals. Washington, DC. December.

Congressional Budget Office. 2009. A preliminary analysis of the President's budget and an update of CBO's Budget and Economic Outlook. Washington, DC. March.

Conover, Christopher J., and Frank A Sloan. 1998. Does removing certificate -of-need regulation lead to a surge in health care spending? *Journal of Health Politics, Policy and Law* 23 (3): 455–81.

Consumer Reports. 2009. Hospital rankings for chronic care. http://www.consumerreports.org/health/doctors-and-hospitals/hospital-home.htm?resultPageIndex=1&resultIndex=1.

Consumers Union. 2003. How good are your state's nursing homes? *Nursing Home Watch List*, June.

Consumer Union. 2009. U.S. health care system fails to protect patients from deadly medical errors. CU Report on Safe Patient Project. May 19. http://www.safepatientproject.org/2009/05/cu_report_us_health_care_syste.html.

Cooper, Michael H. 1975. *Rationing Health Care*. London: Croom Helm.

Council of Economic Advisors. 2009. *Economic Report of the President*. Washington, DC: Government Printing Office.

Cowen, Tyler. 2008. Means testing for Medicare. *New York Times*, July 20: BU N.

Croasdale, Myrle. 2006. Innovative funding opens new residency slots. American Medical Association, January 30. http://www.ama-assn.org/amednews/site/free/prl20130.htm.

Cutler, David M., and Ellen Meara. 2009. Medical costs of the young and old: A forty-year perspective. In *Frontiers in the Economics of Aging*, ed. David A. Wise. Cambridge, MA: National Bureau of Economic Research.

Cutler, David M., and Mark McClellan. 2001. Is technological change in medicine worth it? *Health Affairs* 20 (5): 11–29.

Cutler, David M., J. Bradford Delong, and Ann Marie Marciarille. 2008. Why Obama's health plan is better. *Wall Street Journal*, September 16: 18–19. http://www. online.wsj.com/article/SB122152292213639569.html?mod=googlenews_wsj.

Cutler, David. 2004. *Your Money Or Your Life*. Cambridge: Oxford University Press.

Dalmia, Shikha. 2007. The UAW's health care dreams. *Wall Street Journal*, July 27: A13.

Daschle, Tom. 2008. *Critical: What Can We Do about the Health Care Crisis*. New York: Dunne/St. Martin's Press.

Davis, Karen, et al. 2005. Health and productivity among U.S. workers. Issue Brief 856. The Commonwealth Fund, New York, August.

Davis, Karen. 2008. Slowing the growth of health care costs—Learning from international experience. *New England Journal of Medicine* 359 (17): 1751–55.

Deloitte Center for Health Solutions. 2008. *Medical Tourism: Consumers in Search of Value*. Washington, DC: Deloitte.

Department of Health and Human Services. 2007. An overview of the U.S. Health Care System Chart Book. Centers for Medicare and Medicaid Services, Office of the Assistant Secretary for Planning and Evaluation, Washington, DC.

Department of Health and Human Services. 2009. Medicare and you. Centers for Medicare and Medicaid Services, Washington, DC.

Derbyshire, Robert C. 1969. *Medical Licensure and Discipline in the United States*. Baltimore: Johns Hopkins University Press.

Diamond, Frank. 2001. Blueprint for the future? Or trapped in a lockbox? *Managed Care Magazine*, January. http://www.managedcaremag.com/archives/0101/0101.fehbp.html.

Didion Joan. 2005. The case of Theresa Schiavo. New York Review of Books 52 (10). http://www.nybooks.com/articles/18050.

Ding, Danaei G., Eric L. Ding, Dariush Mozaffarian, Ben Taylor, Jürgen Rehm, Christopher J. L. Murray, and Majid Ezzati. 2009. The preventable causes of death in the United States: Comparative risk assessment of dietary, lifestyle, and metabolic risk factors. *Public Library of Science–Medicine.* http://www.ncbi.nlm.nih.gov/pubmed/19399161?dopt==Abstract.

Dobias, Matthew. 2009. Healthcare opinion leaders survey. *Modern Healthcare,* January 19: 18–19.

Dubay, Lisa, John Holahan, and Allison Cook. 2006. The uninsured and the affordability of health insurance coverage. *Health Affairs* 10. http://www.content.healthaffairs.org/cgi/content/abstract/hlthaff.26.1.w22v1 (downloaded April 23, 2009).

Economist, The. 2008. Idlers under attack. August 30: 52.

Economist, The. 2009a. Medicine goes digital. A special report on health care and technology. April 18: 3–18.

Economist, The. 2009b. The government's finances: Brave rhetoric, grim reality. February 28: 31–32.

Economist, The. 2009c. Life is expensive: Treating the sickest part of America's economy. A Special Report on Business in America. May 30: 12–14.

Edelstein, Ludwig. 1943. *The Hippocratic Oath: Text, Translation and Interpretation.* Baltimore: Johns Hopkins University Press.

Edwards, Chris, and Tad DeHaven. 2003. War between the generations. Policy Analysis 48. Cato Institute, Washington, DC. September 16.

Edwards, Chris, and Jagadeesh Gokhale. 2006. Unfunded state and local health costs: $1.4 trillion. Tax and Budget Bulletin 40. Cato Institute, Washington, DC. October

Eisenberg, David, et al. 1998. Trends in alternative medicine use in the United States, 1990–1997. *Journal of the American Medical Association* 280 (18): 1569–75.

ElderWeb. 2009. Why do we have medicare Part A and Part B? http://www.lderweb.com/home/node/1011.

Elmendorf, Douglas W. 2009. *Expanding Health Insurance Coverage and Controlling Costs for Health Care.* Testimony before the Committee of the Budget. U.S. Senate, February 10. Washington, DC: Congressional Budget Office.

Emanuel, Ezekial, et al. 2003. The cost of conducting clinical research. *Journal of Clinical Oncology* 21 (22): 4145–50.

Emanuel, Ezekial J. 2008. *Healthcare, Guaranteed.* New York: Public Affairs.

Enthoven, Alain. 2008. Health care with a few bucks left over. *New York Times,* December 28 (Op Ed): 9WK.

Evans, Robert G., Morris L. Barer, and Theodore R. Marmor, eds. 1994. *Why Are Some People Healthy And Others Are Not?* New York: Aldine De Gruyter.

Ezzati, Majid. 2004. How can cross-country research on health risks strengthen interventions? Lessons from INTERHEART. *Lancet* 364 (9438): 912–14.

FBI (Federal Bureau of Investigation) 2007. Financial crimes report to the public, fiscal year 2007. http://www.fbi.gov/publications/financial/fcs_rep ort2007/financial_crime_2007.html.

Feldstein, Paul J. 2007. *Health Policy Issues*, 4th ed. Chicago: Health Administration Press.

Feldstein, Martin. 2009. Obama care is all about rationing. *Wall Street Journal*, August 19 (Op Ed): A15.

Filmer, Deon, and Lant Pritchett. 2004. Child mortality and public spending on health: How much does money matter? Policy research working paper 1864. World Bank, Washington, DC. November 14.

Finfacts Ireland Business and Finance Portal. 2007. Going sick to work or staying home healthy?—How national sickness-leave regulations affect workplace absences, June 8. http://www.finfacts.com/irelandbusinessnews/publish/printer_1000article_1010288s .html.

Fisher, Elliott S., David Goodman, Jonathan Skinner, and Kristen Bronner. 2008. Health care spending, quality, and outcomes: More isn't always better. A Dartmouth Atlas Project Topic Brief, February 27. Dartmouth Institute for Health Policy and Clinical Practice, Hanover.

Flood, Colleen, Mark Stabile, and Carolyn Hughes Tuohy. 2008. Introduction. Seeking the grail: Financing for quality, accessability, and sustainability in the health care system. In *Exploring Social Insurance: Can a Dose of Europe Cure Canadian Health Care Finance?* eds. Colleen M. Flood, Mark Stabile, and Carolyn Hughes Tuohy. Montreal: McGill-Queen's University Press, 1–36.

Fox News, 2009. Universal health care may cost $1.5 trillion. http://www.foxnews.com/ politics/first100days/2009/18/universal-health-care-cost-trillion.

Fox, Will, and John Pickering. 2008. *Hospital and Physician Cost Shift: Payment Level Comparison of Medicare, Medicaid, and Commercial Payers*. Seattle, WA: Milliman Consulting.

Freelancers Union. 2009. Insurance. http://www.freelancersunion.org/insurance.

Freidson, Eliot. 1970. *Profession of Medicine*. Chicago: University of Chicago Press.

Friedlander, Robert B. 2005. Insuring real life. *Generations: Journal of the American Society on Aging*. http://www.asaging.org/generations/gen29-1/article_insuringreallife.cfm.

Fronstin, Paul. 2001. Sources of health insurance and characteristics of the uninsured: Analysis of the March 2001 Current Population Survey. EBRI Issue Brief 240. Employee Benefit Research Institute, Washington, DC.

Fronstin, Paul. 2007a. Sources of health insurance and characteristics of the uninsured: An analysis of the March 2007 Current Population Survey. EBRI Issue Brief 310. Employee Benefit Research Institute, Washington, DC.

Fronstin, Paul. 2007b. The future of employment-based health benefits: Have employers reached a tipping point? EBRI Issue Brief 312. Employee Benefit Research Institute, Washington, DC.

Fronstin, Paul, and Dallas Salisbury. 2007. Health insurance and taxes: Can changing the tax treatment of health insurance fix our health care system? EBRI Issue Brief 309. Employee Benefit Research Institute, Washington, DC.

Fronstin, Paul. 2008a. Findings from the 2008 EBRI Consumer Engagement in Health Care Survey. EBRI Issue Brief 323. Employee Benefit Research Institute, Washington, DC.

Fronstin, Paul. 2008b. The impact of immigration on health insurance coverage in the United States, 1994–2006. Employee Benefit Research Institute. *EBRI Notes* 29 (8): 3–12.

Fronstin, Paul, and Stephen Blakely. 2008. Is the tipping point near? *Wall Street Journal*, April 22: A16.

Fronstin, Paul. 2009. Capping the tax exclusion for employment-based health coverage: Implications for employers and workers. Executive Summary. EBRI Issue Brief 325. Employee Benefit Research Institute, Washington, DC.

Fuchs, Victor R. 1972. The contribution of health services to the American economy. In *Essays in the Economics of Health and Medical Care*, ed. Victor R. Fuchs. New York: Columbia University Press, 3–38.

Fuchs, Victor R. 1981. Economics, health, and post-industrial society. In *Economics and Health Care*, ed. John B. McKinlay. Cambridge: MIT Press, 1–30.

Fuchs, Victor R. 2008. Three inconvenient truths about health care. *New England Journal of Medicine* 359 (17): 1749–51.

Fuhrmans, Vanessa. 2008. Insurers stop paying for care linked to errors. *Wall Street Journal*, January 15: D1.

Gaffney, Declan, Allyson M. Pollock, and Jean Shaoul. 1999. NHS capital expenditure and the private finance initiative: Expansion or contraction? *British Medical Journal* 319: 48–51.

Galbraith, John Kenneth, and Nicole Salinger. 1978. *Almost Everyone's Guide to Economics*. Mount Vernon, NY: Consumers Union.

Galbraith, John Kenneth. 1958. *The Affluent Society*. Boston: Houghton Mifflin.

Gale, William G., and Alan J. Auerbach. 2009. *Here Comes the Next Fiscal Crisis.*Washington, DC: Brookings Institution.

Galvin, Robert S. 2008. Still in the game: Harnessing employer inventiveness in U.S. health care reform. *New England Journal of Medicine* 359 (14): 1421–23.

Garber, Alan M., and Jonathan Skinner. 2008. Is American health care uniquely inefficient? Journal of Economic Perspectives 22 (4): 27–50.

Garber, Alan M., and Jonathan Skinner. 2008. Is American health care uniquely inefficient? Working paper W14257. National Bureau of Economic Research, Cambridge, MA.

Gautam Naik. 2008. The toughest test and more prenatal testing brings new worries. *Wall Street Journal*, October 25: A1.

Georgetown University Health Policy Institute. 2007. Long-*Term Care Financing Project, National Spending for Long-Term Care Fact Sheet*. Washington, DC: Georgetown University.

Ginsberg, Paul, and Joy M. Grossman. 2005. When the price isn't right: How inadvertent payment incentives drive medical care. *Health Affairs*. Health Tracking: Marketwatch, August 9. http://www.content.healthaffairs.org/cgi/content/full/hlthaff.w5.376/DC1.

Gorsky, Martin. 2008. The British National Health Service 1948–2008: A review of the historiography. *Social History of Medicine* 21 (3): 437–60.

Gould, Elsie. 2004. Health care: U.S. spends more, gets less. Snapshots Archive. Economic Policy Institute, Washington, DC. October 20.

Greenspan, Alan. 2007. *The Age of Turbulence*. New York: Penguin.

Gross, Jane. 2008. AIDS patients face downside of living longer. *New York Times*, January 6: 1, 12.

Gruber, John. 2006. *The Role of Consumer Co-payments for Health care: Lessons from the RAND Health Insurance Experiment and Beyond*. Menlo Park, CA: Kaiser Family Foundation.

Gruber, Jonathan. 2002. Rising unemployment and the uninsured. Kaiser Family Foundation, January. http://www.kff.org/uninsured/7850.cfm.

Gruber, Jonathan. 2009. Universal health insurance coverage or economic relief: A false choice. *New England Journal of Medicine* 360 (1): 437–39.

Guttmacher Institute. 2008. In brief: Facts on induced abortion in the United States, July. http://www.guttmacher.org/pubs/fb_induced_abortion.html.

Guttmacher Institute. 2008. Media center: U.S. abortion rate continues long-term decline, falling to lowest level since 1974; more effort still needed to reduce unintended pregnancy, January 17. http://www.guttmacher.org/media/nr/2008/01/17/index.html.

Hampson, Lindsay A., and Ezekial J. Emanuel. 2005. The prognosis for changes in end-of-life care after the Schiavo case. *Health Affairs* 24 (4): 972–75.

Harris, Richard. 1966. *A Sacred Trust*. New York: New American Library.

HealthGrades. 2009. Latest HealthGrade studies. http://www.healthgrades.com/.

Hechinger, John. 2009. Court rules on funding special education. *Wall Street Journal*, June 23: A4.

Helrman, Ruth, et al. 2009. The 2009 Retirement Confidence Survey: Economy drives confidence to record low; many looking to work longer. Issue Brief 328. Employee Benefit Research Institute, Washington, DC.

Henry J. Kaiser Family Foundation. 2004. Current trends and future outlook for retiree health benefits: Findings from the Kaiser/Hewitt 2004 Survey on Retiree Health Benefits. http://www.kff.org/medicare/med121404pkg.cfm.

Henry J. Kaiser Family Foundation. 2007. Snapshots: Health care costs, how changes in medical technology affect health care costs. http://www.kff.org/insurance/snapshot/chcm030807oth.cfm.

Herlinger, Regina. 1997. *Market Driven Health Care*. Reading, MA: Addison-Wesley.

Herrick, Devon M. 2005. Crisis of the uninsured: 2005 update. Brief Analysis 528. National Center for Policy Analysis, Washington, DC. September 22.

1994. Hertzman, Clyde, John Frank, and Robert G. Evans. 1994. Heterogeneities in health status and the determinants of population health. In *Why Are Some People Healthy and Others Not?* eds. Robert G. Evans, Morris L. Barer, and Theodore R. Marmor. New York: Aldine De Gruyter, 67–92.

Herzlinger, Regina. 2007. *Who Killed Health Care?* New York: McGraw-Hill.

Himmelstein, David U., et al. 1999. Quality of care in investor-owned vs not-for-profit HMOs. *Journal of the American Medical Association* 282 (2): 159–63.

Himmelstein, David U., and Steffie Woolhandler. 2003. National health insurance or incremental reform: Aim high, or at our feet. *American Journal of Public Health* 93 (1): 102–105.

Hodges, Michael. 2009. Grandfather federal government debt report summary page. http://www.home.att.net/~mwhodges/debt.html (accessed March 13, 2009).

Hudson, Robert P. 1978. Abraham Flexner in perspective: American medical education 1865–1910. In *Sickness and Health in America*, eds. Judith Walzer Levitt and Ronald L. Numbers. Madison: University of Wisconsin Press, 105–15.

Iglehart, John K. 2008. Medicare, graduate medical education, and new policy directions. *New England Journal of Medicine* 359 (6): 643–50.

Iglehart, John K. 2009a. The struggle for reform: Challenges and hopes for comprehensive health care legislation. *New England Journal of Medicine* 360 (17): 1693–95.

Iglehart, John K. 2009b. Prioritizing comparative-effectiveness research: IOM recommendations. *New England Journal of Medicine* 360 (4): 325–28.

Illich, Ivan. 1975. *Medical Nemesis*. London: Calder and Boyars.

Institute of Medicine. 2000. *To Err Is Human: Building a Safer Health System*. Washington, DC: National Academy Press.

International Task Force on Euthanasia and Assisted Suicide. 2008. Failed attempts to legalize euthanasia/assisted suicide. http://www.Internationaltaskforce.org/usa.html.

Jencks, Stephen F., Mark V. Williams, and Eric A. Coleman. 2009. Rehospitalizations among patients in the Medicare fee-for-service program. *New England Journal of Medicine* 360 (14): 1418–28.

Kahn, James G., Richard Kronick, Mary Krager, and David N. Gans. 2005. The cost of health insurance administration in California: Estimates for insurers, physicians and hospitals. *Health Affairs* 24 (6): 1629–39.

Kennedy, Dennis, Scoll Clay, and Deborah Kolb Collier. 2009. Factors driving the physician employment trend. *Healthcare Financial Magazine*. Healthcare Financial Management Association. April. http://www.hfma.org/hfm/2009archives/month04/HFM0409web exclusive_kennedy.html.

Kirkegaard, Funk. 2009. Europe and the US: Whose health care is more socialistic? New York: Peterson Institute for International Economics. http://www.piie.com/realtime/?p=595 (accessed September 1, 2009).

Klarman, Herbert E. 1965. *The Economics of Health*. New York: Columbia University Press.

Kling, Arnold. 2006. *Crisis of Abundance: Rethinking How We Pay for Health Care*. Washington, DC: Cato Institute.

Knaus, William A. 1981. *Inside Russian Medicine*. New York: Everest House.

Knight, Al. 2000. Immigration and the uninsured. Center for Immigration Studies. *Denver Post*, September 24. http://www.cis.org/articles/2000/coverage/newscoverage.html.

Knowledge@EmorySeptember. 2003. The mounting challenge of bringing a drug to market. http://www.knowledge.emory.edu/article.cfm?articleid=718.

Kotlikoff, Laurence J., and Scott Burns. 2004. *The Coming Generational Storm: What You Need to Know about America's Economic Future*. Cambridge: MIT Press.

Kronick, Richard. 2009. Medicare and HMOs: The search for accountability. *New England Journal of Medicine* 360 (20): 2048–50.

Krugman, Paul, and Robin Wells. The health care crisis and what to do about it. *New York Review of Books* 53 (5). http://www.nybooks.com/articles/18802.

Kuttner, Robert. 1998. Must good HMOs go bad? The commercialization of prepaid group health care. First of two parts. *New England Journal of Medicine*. 338 (21): 1558–63; and part II 338 (22): 1635–39.

Landro, Laura. 2005. The informed patient. *Wall Street Journal*, March 9: D9.

Le Fanu, James. 1999. *The Rise and Fall of Modern Medicine*. New York: Carrol and Graf.

Leapfrog Group, The. 2009. http://www.leapfroggroup.org/about_us/other_initiatives/incentives_and_rewards/bridges_to_excellence.

Lee, Thomas H., and Ezekial J. Emanuel. 2008. Tier 4 drugs and the fraying of the social compact. *New England Journal of Medicine* 359 (4): 333–35.

Lewis, Hunter. 2007. *Are the Rich Necessary?* Mount Jackson, VA: Axios Press.

Lo, Bernard, and Marilyn J. Field, eds. 2009. *Conflict of Interest in Medical Research, Education, and Practice*. Washington, DC: National Academy Press.

Locke, Gary. 2009. Fixing health care is good for business. *Wall Street Journal*, August 28 (Op Ed): A13.

Lowenstein, Roger. 2008. *While America Aged*. New York: Penguin.

Lubitz, James D., and Gerald F. Riley. 1993. Trends in Medicare payments in the last year of life. *New England Journal of Medicine* 328 (15): 1092–96.

Lyke, Bob. 2008. The tax exclusion for employer-provided health insurance: Policy issues regarding the repeal debate. Report to Congress. Congressional Research Service, Washington, DC. November 21.

MakeThemAccountable. 2008. http://www.makethemaccountable.com/myth/RisingCostOfMedicalMalpracticeInsurance.html.

Mankiw, Gregory N. 2007. Beyond those health care numbers. *New York Times*, November 4 (Sunday issue, Economic View column): 4.

Marks, Alexandra. 2009. Healthcare battle brewing: Politicians gear up. *Christian Science Monitor*, April 8. http://www.features.csmonitor.com/politics/2009/04/08/healthcare-battle-brewing-political-groups-gear-up.

Martinez, Barbara, and John Carreyrou. 2009. Minority of tax-exempt hospitals provide most charity care. *Wall Street Journal*, February 13: A3.

Matthews, Merrill. 2006. Medicare's hidden administrative costs: A comparison of Medicare and the private sector. Council for Affordable Health Insurance, January 10. http://www.cahi.org/cahi_contents/resources/pdf/CAHI_Medicare_Admin_Final_Publication.pdf.

McCormack, Lauren A., Jon R. Gabel, Heidi Whitmore, Wayne L. Anderson, and Jeremy Pickreign. 2002. Trends in retiree health benefits. *Health Affairs* 21 (6): 169–76.

McKeown, Thomas. 1976. *The Role of Medicine*. London: Nuffield Provincial Hospitals Trust.

McKinlay, John B., and Sonja M. McKinlay. 1980. The questionable contribution of medical measures to the decline of mortality in the United States in the twentieth century. In *Issues in Health Services*, ed. Stephen J. Williams. New York: Wiley, 3–16.

McKinsey Global Institute. 2008. Accounting for the Cost of US health care: A new look at why Americans spend more, November. http://www.mckinsey.com/mgi/publications/US_healthcare.

McQueen, M. P. Health insurers target the individual market. *Wall Street Journal*, August 21: D1, D3.

McTague, Jim. 2006. The trillion-dollar pothole. *Barrons Magazine*, March 13. http://www.barrons.com/article/SB117693814485374763.html?mod.

Mechanic, David. 2000. Managed care and the imperative for a new professional ethic. *Health Affairs* 19 (5): 100–11.

Mechanic, David. 2006. *The Truth about Health Care*. New Brunswick: Rutgers University Press.

Medicare Payment Advisory Commission. 2003. Relationships among Medicare inpatient, overall Medicare and total margins for hospitals. Medicare Payment Advisory Commission (MEDPAC), Washington, DC. August. http://www.medpac.gov/publications/other_reports/Aug03_hosp_marg_2pgr_AW.pdf (accessed August 7, 2003).

Mehlman, Maxwell J. 2005.Off-label prescribing. The doctor will see you now, May. http://www.thedoctorwillseeyounow.com/articles/bioethics/offlabel_11/.

Merritt, David, ed. 2007. *Paper Kills: Transforming Health and Healthcare with Information Technology*. Washington, DC: CHT Press.

Michaud, Catherine M., et al. 2001. Burden of disease: Implications for future research. *Journal of the American Medical Association* 285 (5): 535–39.

Milbank Memorial Fund, National Association of State Budget Officers, and Reforming States Group. 2005. 2002–2003 State Health Expenditure Report, June. http://www.Milbank.org/reports/05NASBO/index.html.

Millenson, Michael L. 1997. *Demanding Medical Excellence*. Chicago: University of Chicago Press.

Miller, Robert, and Ida Sim. 2004. Physicians' use of electronic medical records: Barriers and solutions. *Health Affairs* 23 (2): 116–26.

Moore, Jonathan, and J. Duncan Jr. 2000. HCFA moving on anesthesia rule. *Modern Healthcare* 30 (12): 14.

Moses, Stephen A. 2005. Aging America's Achilles' heel Medicaid long-term care. Policy Analysis 549. Cato Institute, Washington, DC. September 1.

National Association of State Budget Officers. 2002. NASBO analysis: Medicaid to stress state budgets severely into fiscal 2003. March 15.

National Coalition on Health Care. 2009. Health insurance costs. http://www.nchc.org/facts/cost.shtml.

National Conference of State Legislatures. 2008. Managed care and health insurance state laws for ombudsman, report cards and provider profiles. May. http://www.ncsl.org/programs/health/hmorep2.htm.

National Council Against Health Fraud. 2002. NCAHF position statement on White House Commission on Complementary and Alternative Medicine, March 25. http://www.quackwatch.org/01QuackeryRelatedTopics/whcpp.html.

National Governors' Association. 2008. Economic stimulus, state budget shortfalls, and state countercyclical funding. http://www.nga.org/files/pdf/0801stimulusinformation.pdf.

National Health Care Anti-Fraud Association. 2009. The problem of health care fraud. Anti-Fraud Resource Center. http://www.nhcaa.org/eweb/DynamicPage.aspx?webcode=anti_fraud_resource_centr&wpscode=TheProblemOfHCFraud (accessed April 9, 2009).

New York Academy of Medicine. 1958. Origins of the cost problem. In *Readings in Medical Care*, ed. Committee on Medicare Teaching. Chapel Hill: University of North Carolina Press, 115–17.

Newhouse, Joseph. 1992. Medical care costs: How much welfare loss? *Journal of Economic Perspectives* 6 (3): 3–21.

Newhouse, Joseph P. 2004. Consumer-directed health plans and the Rand health insurance experiment. *Health Affairs* 23 (6): 107–13.

Nixon, Joseph. 2008. Why doctors are headed for Texas. *Wall Street Journal*, May 17: A9.

O'Sullivan, Jennifer. 2008. Medicare: History of Part A Trust Fund Insolvency Projections. Report for Congress. Congressional Research Service, Washington, DC. March 28.

Organization for Economic Cooperation and Development. 2005. Ageing populations: High time for action. Meeting of G8 Employment and Labour Ministers. March 10–11. London. http://www.oecd.org/LongAbstract/0,3425,en_2649_201185_34600620_1_1_1_1,00.html.

Organization for Economic Cooperation and Development. 2006. OECD health data 2006. http://www.oecd.org/dataoecd/29/52/36960035.

Orszag, Peter R. 2008a. Increasing the value of federal health spending on health care. Testimony before the Committee on the Budget. US House of Representatives. July 16.

Orszag, Peter R. 2008b. New ideas about human behavior in economics and medicine. Eighth Annual Marshall J. Seidman Lecture. Harvard Medical School. Washington, DC: Congressional Budget Office.

Orszag. Peter R. 2008c. The overuse, underuse, and misuse of health care. Testimony before the U.S. Senate Committee on Finance. Washington, DC: Congressional Budget Office. July 17.

Parsons, Talcott. 1979. Definitions of health and illness in the light of American values ND social structure. In *Patients, Physicians and Illness*, ed. E. Gartly Jaco. New York: Free Press.

Paterson, Craig. 2004. Health care, social justice and the common good, April 19. SSRN. http://www.ssrn.com/abstract=1097135.

Pauly, Mark V. 1988. Is medical care different? Old questions, new answers. *Journal of Health Politics, Policy and Law* 13 (2): 227–37.

PBS Frontline. 2003. The Alternate Fix, November 6. http://www.pbs.org/wgbh/pages/frontline/shows/altmed/etc/synopsis.html.

Pear, Robert. 2008a. Budget Office sees hurdles in financing health plans. *New York Times*, December 19: A28.

Pear, Robert. 2008b. When a job disappears, so does the health care. *New York Times*. December 8 (Sunday issue): 30N

Penner, Rudolph G., and Julianna Koch. 2007. *How Much Spending Is Uncontrollable?* Washington, DC: Urban Institute. http://www.urban.org/publications/1001093.html (accessed July 16, 2007).

Penner, Rudolph G., and C. Eugene Steurle. 2009. *Budget Crisis at the Door*. Washington, DC: Urban Institute. http://www.urban.org/publications/310883.html (accessed October 1, 2009).

Perry, Mark J. 2008. Carpe diem, the crippling burden of legacy costs: GM is a health care company that sells cars on the side. http://www.mjperry.blogspot.com/2008/11/crippling-burden-of-legacy-costs-gm-is.html (accessed March 10, 2009).

Peter, G. Peterson Foundation. 2009. *Issues: National Economic Responsibility*. http://www.pgpf.org/issues/fiscalresponsibility (accessed April 22, 2009).

Peterson, Chris L., and Rachel Burton. 2007. U.S. health care spending: Comparison with other OECD countries. Report to Congress. Congressional Research Service, Washington, DC. September 17.

Peterson, Peter G. 2004. *Running on Empty*. New York: Farrar, Straus and Giroux.

Pew Center on the States. 2006. *Special Report on Medicaid*. Philadelphia: Pew Charitable Trusts.

Physicians for a National Health Program. 2006. Medical-loss ratios of largest for-profit insurers. March 20. http://www.pnhp.org/news/2006/march/medalloss_ratios_.php.

Physicians for a National Health Program. 2007. Single payer national health insurance. http://www.pnhp.org/facts/single_payer_resources.php (accessed December 19, 2007).

Picker, Randal C. 2008. The legal infrastructure of business: Health insurance consolidation. http://www.picker.typepad.com/legal_infrastructure_of_b/2008/12/health-insurance-consolidation.html (accessed December 1, 2008).

Pierron, William, and Paul Fronstin. 2008. ERISA Pre-emption: Implications for Health Reform. Employee Benefit Research Institute. EBRI Issue Brief 314. February.

Pipes, Sally C. 2009. Health 'reformers' ignore fact. *Wall Street Journal*, March 6: A15.

Pollack, Allyson M. 2004. *The Privatization of Free Care*. London: Verso.

Porter, Michael E. and Teisberg, Elizabeth Olmsted. 2004. Redefining competition in health care. *Harvard Business Review OnPoint*. Product 696.

Practice Management Resources Medical Group Management Association. 2004. Date derived from 2004 MGMA Study of MGMA members. Provided by personal communication with David Gans, Vice President, December 9.

Practice Management Resources Medical Group Management Association. 2005. Estimates for the distribution of medical groups and physicians. Provided by personal communication with David Gans, Vice President, December 10.

President's Commission for the Study of Ethical Problems in Medicine and Biomedical and Behavioral Research. 1983. *Securing Access to Health Care. Volume 1: The Ethical Implications of Differences in the Availability of Health Services.* Washington, DC: Government Printing Office.

PriceWaterhouseCoopers. 2005. Health Cast 2000: Creating a sustainable future. Health Research Institute. http://www.eucomed.org/upload/pdf/tl/2005/extranet/communications/resources/healthcast2020.pdf.

PriceWaterhouseCoopers. 2006. My brother's keeper: Growing expectations confront hospitals on community benefits and charity care. Health Research Institute. http://www.pwc.com/extweb/pwcpublications.nsf/docid/38BE1BA9F194D10F85257308005936AB.

PriceWaterhouseCoopers. 2009. A global look at balancing demand, quality, and efficiency in healthcare payment reform. http://www.pwc.com/extweb/pwcpublications.nsf/docid/BC589DEBA59D9B228525746500600790 (accessed February 1, 2009).

Public Citizen. 2006. Ranking of state medical board serious disciplinary actions: 2003–2005. Health Research Group Publication 1766. http://www.citizen.org/publications/release.cfm?ID=7428&secID=1158&catID=126.

Radley, David C., Stan N. Finkelstein, and Randall S. Stafford. 2006. Off-label prescribing among office-based physicians. *Archives of Internal Medicine* 166 (9): 1021–26.

Raffel, Marshall W., ed. 1985. *Comparative Health Systems.* University Park: Pennsylvania State University Press.

Rand Corporation. 2009. Health information technology: Can HIT lower costs and improve quality? Rand Corporation Research Briefs. http://www.rand.org/pubs/research_briefs/RB9136/index1.html.

Rappaport, Liz. 2009. Rescue efforts ding U.S.'s triple-A rating. *Wall Street Journal,* February 13: C2.

Reports, Rasmussen. 2009. Social Security: 46% favor opting out of Social Security. http://www.rasmussenreports.com/public_content/politics/mood_of_america/social_security/social_security.

Reeves, Laurant M., et al. 2004. Substitution of doctors by nurses in primary care. Cochrane Database of Systematic Reviews (Online:Update Software), Issue 4: CD001271. doi:10.1002/14651858.CD001271.pub2.

Reid, T. R. 2009. *The Healing of America: A Global Quest for Better, Cheaper, and Fairer Health Care.* New York: Penguin.

Reinhardt, Uwe E., Peter S. Hussey, and Gerard F. Anderson. 2004. U.S. health care spending in an international context. *Health Affairs* 23 (3): 10–25.

Relman, Arnold. 1980. The new medical-industrial complex. *New England Journal of Medicine* 303 (17): 963–70.

Relman, Arnold. 2007. *A Second Opinion: Rescuing America's Health Care.* Cambridge, MA: Public Affairs.

Rice, Thomas. 1997. *The Case for Universal Health Coverage in the Future U.S. Healthcare System: Who Will Care for the Poor and Uninsured?* eds. Stuart H. Altman, Uwe E. Reinhardt, and Alexandra E. Shields. Chicago: Health Administration Press.

Richmond, Julius B., and Rashi Fein. 2005. *The Health Care Mess.* Cambridge: Harvard University Press.

Robinson, James C. 2004a. Consolidation and the transformation of competition in health insurance. *Health Affairs* 23 (6): 11–24.

Robinson, James C. 2004b. Interview: Business opportunities in transforming health care. A conversation with William W. McGuire. *Health Affairs* 23 (6): 114–21.

Roemer, Milton I., ed. 1960. *Henry E. Sigerist on the Sociology of Medicine.* New York: MD Publications.

Romano, Michael. 2005. Perception is everything. *Modern Healthcare* 35 (10): 6–7, 13.

Roscoe, Lori A., and Thomas J. Krizek. 2002. Reporting medical errors. *Bulletin of the American College of Surgeons* 87 (9): 12–17.

Rosenbaum, Sara, D. Richard Mauery, Peter Shin, and Julia Hidalgo. 2005. National Security and U.S. child health policy: The origins and continuing role of Medicaid and EPSDT. Policy Brief. George Washington School of Public Health and Health Services, Department of Health Policy, Washington, DC.

Russell, Louise B. 2009. Preventing chronic disease: An important investment, but don't count on cost savings. *Health Affairs* 28 (1): 42–45.

Rutledge, Robert. 1998. An analysis of 25 Milliman and Robertson guidelines for surgery. *Annals of Surgery* 228 (4): 579–87.

Sack, Kevin. 2008. Necessary medicine? Health care and the economy share a sickbed. Maybe they can recover together. *New York Times*, December 14 (Sunday issue): 1, 4WK.

Samuelson, Robert J. 2008. *The Great Inflation and Its Aftermath.* New York: Random House.

Schneider, Eric, Alan Zaslavsky, and Arnold Epstein. 2005. Quality of care in for-profit and not-for-profit health plans enrolling Medicare beneficiaries. *American Journal of Medicine* 118 (12): 1392–1400.

Sherlock Company. 2008. Blues post modest trends in administrative costs in 2007. Plan Management Navigator, July. http://www.sherlockco.com/docs/navigator/navigator -08-07.pdf.

Shi, Leiyu, and Douglas A. Singh. 2008. *Delivering Health Care in America: A Systems Approach.* Boston: Jones and Bartlett.

Shryock, Richard Harrison. 1967. *Medical Licensing in America, 1650–1965.* Baltimore: Johns Hopkins University Press.

Sloan, Frank A. 2000. Not-for-profit ownership and hospital behavior. In *Handbook of Health Economics*, eds. Anthony J. Culyer and Joseph P. Newhouse. New York: Elsevier.

Social Security Administration. 2009. Actuarial publications. Status of the Social Security and Medicare Programs. Summary of the 2009 Annual Reports. Social Security online. http://www.ssa.gov/OACT/TRSUM/index.html (accessed May 14, 2009).

Sparer, Michael. 2009. Medicaid and the U.S. path to national health insurance. *New England Journal of Medicine* 360 (4): 323–25.

Sparrow, Malcom K. 1996. *License to Steal: Why Fraud Plagues America's Health Care System.* Boulder, CO: Westview Press.

Sparrow, Malcom K. 2009. Criminal prosecution as a deterrent to health care fraud. Testimony before the Senate Judiciary Subcommittee on Crime and Drugs, Washington, DC. May 20.

Stafford, Randall S. 2008. Regulating off-label drug use: Rethinking the role of the FDA. *New England Journal of Medicine* 358 (14): 1427–29.

Starfield, Barbara. 2000. Is U.S. health care really the best in the world? *Journal of the American Medical Association* 284: 483–85.

Starr, Paul. 1982. *The Social Transformation of American Medicine.* New York: Basic Books.

Stephen, William John. 1979. *An Analysis of Primary Medical Care: An International Study.* New York: Cambridge University Press.

Stoll, John D. 2009. GM nears crucial deal with UAW. *Wall Street Journal,* May 15: B1, B2.

Styring, William, III, and Donald K. Jonas. 1999. *Health Care 2020: The Coming Collapse of Employer-Provided Health Care.* Indianapolis: Hudson Institute.

Terhune, Chad, Keith Epstein, and Catherine Arnst. 2009. The dubious promise of digital medicine. *Business Week,* May 4: 31–37.

Thaler, Richard H., and Cass R. Sunstein. 2008. *Nudge: Improving Decisions about Health, Wealth, and Happiness.* New Haven: Yale University Press.

Thompson, Lindsay A., David C. Goodman, and George A. Little. 2002. Is more neonatal intensive care always better? Insights from a cross-national comparison of reproductive care. *Pediatrics* 109 (6): 1036–43.

Thomson, Sarah, and Elias Mossialos. 2008. Medical savings accounts: Can they improve health system performance in Europe? *Euro Observer* 10 (4): 1–6.

Times Online. 2006. NHS must audit spending on alternative therapy, MPs say, May 24. http://www.timesonline.co.uk/tol/life_and_style/health/alternative_medicine/article 724775.ece.

Torres, Aida, Patricia Donovan, Nancy Dittes, and Jacqueline D. Forrest. 1986. Public benefits and costs of government funding for abortion. *Family Planning Perspectives* 18 (3): 111–18.

Tu, Ha T., and James D. Reschovsky. 2002. Assessments of medical care by enrollees in for-profit and nonprofit health maintenance organizations. *New England Journal of Medicine* 346 (17): 1288–93.

Tufts Center for the Study of Drug Development. 2009. *Research Milestones.* http://www.csdd.tufts.edu/Research/Milestones.asp (accessed April 22, 2009).

Tulchinsky, Theodore H., and Elena A. Varavikova. 2008. *The New Public Health,* 2nd ed. Amsterdam: Elsevier.

Turner, Grace-Marie. 2007. Customer health care. *Wall Street Journal,* May 14: A17.

Turner, Leigh. 2007. Canadian Medicare and the global health bazaar. Policy Options Health File. September. http://www.irpp.org/po/archive/sep07/turner.pdf.

United Health Foundation. 2008. http://www.americashealthrankings.org/2008/other nations.html.

US Department of Health and Human Services, Centers for Medicare and Medicaid Services, and Office of the Assistant Secretary for Planning and Evaluation. 2007. *Overview of the U.S. Health Care System Chart Book*, January 31: table 1.1.

US Department of Health and Human Services. 2006a. National Center for Health Statistics. http://www.cdc.gov/nchs/data/hus/hus06.pdf.

US Department of Health and Human Services. 2006b. *National Nursing Home Survey 2004. Nursing Home Facilities.* December: table 1. National Center for Health Statistics. http://www.cdc.gov/nchs/nnhs.html.

US Department of Health and Human Services. 2008a. A profile of older Americans. Administration on Aging. http://www.aoa.gov/AoAroot/Aging_Statistics/Profile/2007/index.aspx.

US Department of Health and Human Services, and Department of Justice. 2008b. Health care fraud and abuse control program. Annual Report for FY 2007. Washington, DC: Government Printing Office. November.

US Department of Health and Human Services. 2009. Hospital compare a quality tool provided by Medicare. http://www.hospitalcompare.hhs.gov/Hospital/Search?Welcome .asp? (accessed April 26, 2009).

US Department of Labor, and Moynihan Report. 1965. *The Negro Family: The Case for National Action.* Office of Policy Planning and Research. Office of the Assistant Secretary for Administration. Washington, DC: Government Printing Office.

US Government Accountability Office. 2005. Leslie G Aronivitz: Testimony before the Committee on Finance. US Senate Medicaid Fraud and Abuse: CMS's Commitment to helping states safeguard program dollars is limited. Washington, DC, June 28. http://www.gao.gov/new.items/d05855t.pdf.

Verghese, Abraham. 2009. The myth of prevention. *Wall Street Journal*, June 20–21: W1–W2.

Vermeire, Etienne, Hilary Hearnshaw, Paul Van Royen, and Jake Denekens. 2001. Patient adherence to treatment: Three decades of research. A comprehensive review. *Journal of Clinical Pharmacy and Therapeutics* 26 (5):331–442.

Walker, David M. 2008. U.S. financial condition and fiscal future briefing. National Press Foundation. January 17. US Government Accountability Office. GAO-08–446CG.

Walker, Marcus. 2007. Sweden clamps down on sick and disability pay. *Wall Street Journal*, May 9: A1.

Wall Street Journal, The. 2009. The real stimulus burden, February 12.

Walton, Surrey M., Glen T. Schumock, Ky-Van Lee, G. Caleb Alexander, David Meltzer, and Randall S. Stafford. 2008. Prioritizing future research on off-label prescribing. *Pharmacotherapy* 28 (12): 1443–52.

Watson Wyatt National Business Group on Health. 2009a. The one percent strategy: Lessons learned from best performers. http://www.watsonwyatt.com/research/resrender.asp?id=2008-US-0037.

Watson Wyatt National Business Group on Health. 2009b. Employer interest in consumer directed plans growing. Watson Wyatt National Business Group on Health Survey Finds. http://www.watsonwyatt.com/news/press.asp?ID=15826.

Weintraub, Arlene, and Amy Barrett. 2006. Medicine in conflict. Special report. *Business Week*, October 23: 76–87.

Weisman, Jonathan. 2008. Compiling a to-do list for Obama's costly New Deal. *Wall Street Journal*, December 18: A14.

Welch, H. Gilbert, Lisa M. Schwartz, and Steven Woloshin. 2000. Are increasing 5-year survival rates evidence of success against cancer? *Journal of the American Medical Association* 283 (22): 2975–78.

Wennberg, John E., Shannon Brownlee, Elliot S. Fisher, Jonathan S. Skinner, and James N. Weinstein. 2008. Improving quality and curbing health care spending: Opportunities for the Congress and the Obama administration. Dartmouth Atlas White Paper. Dartmouth Institute for Health Policy and Clinical Practice. December.

WHO (World Health Organization). 2002. The role of the private sector and privatization in European health systems. Regional Committee for Europe, 52nd session, Copenhagen, September 16–19. http://www.euro.who.int/Document/RC52/edoc10.pdf.

Wilkinson, Richard, and Kate Pickett. 2009. *The Spirit Level: Why More Equal Societies Almost Always Do Better*. London: Allen Lane.

Wilkinson, Richard G. 1997. Socioeconomic determinants of health: Health inequalities; relative or absolute material standards? *British Medical Journal* 314: 590–94.

Williams, Stephen J., and Paul R. Torrens. 2008. *Introduction to Health Services*, 7th ed. New York: Thomson Delmar Learning.

Woolhandler, Steffie, David U. Himmelstein, and James P. Lewontin. 2003a. Costs of health care administration in the United States and Canada. *New England Journal of Medicine* 349 (8): 768–75.

Woolhandler, Steffie, David U. Himmelstein, Marcia Angell, and Quentin D. Young, Physicians Working Group for Single Payer National Health Insurance. 2003b. Proposal of the physicians' working group for single payer national health insurance. *Journal of the American Medical Association* 290 (6): 798–805.

Zycher, Benjamin. 2009. HAS health-insurance plans after four years: What have we learned? Medical Progress Report 8. http://www.manhattan-institute.org/html/mpr_08.html (accessed February 2009).

Index